Milk

Emma

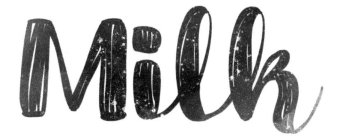

Milk

BY

EMMA ROSEN

A STORY OF
BREASTFEEDING IN A SOCIETY THAT'S
FORGOTTEN HOW.

Sartain Publishing

Published by Sartain Publishing Ltd, London
www.sartainpublishing.co.uk

First edition October 2018
Also available as an eBook

Edited by Kim Kimber
www.kimkimber.co.uk

Cover design and interior formatting by Eight Little Pages
www.eightlittlepages.com

ISBN 978-1-9996292-0-5

For Finlay, Mae and Zoe

CONTENTS

PREFACE

It is dark here in my bedroom. The only light glows dimly from my laptop. As I begin to write these words my twelve-week old baby is sleeping in a Moses basket by my bed. He is overwhelmingly beautiful, peacefully lying there, breathing softly. This little bundle is the centre of my world and my unexpected literary inspiration.

I have always intended to write a book. When I was small I always said I wanted to be an author rather than an astronaut or a princess. As I grew older I started a myriad of tales, only to become disenchanted with the plot all too quickly. I hoped it would simply be a case of finding a subject that gripped me sufficiently to keep me writing, but the right one seemed to elude me.

I knew motherhood would be life-changing and would give me a lot to be passionate about, but I certainly did not expect to find that feeding my baby would reveal a whole world I was completely unaware of. Who would have thought it would be the thing to finally inspire me to start writing?

What authority do I have to write such a book? Who cares about what I have to say? I'm not famous and I'm far from an expert. But I am a mother who has breastfed a baby. Every mother and baby has their own personal tale. This is mine.

ACKNOWLEDGEMENTS

Firstly, I would like to thank Kim Kimber for an interesting and straightforward editing experience. The wonderful design of this book is thanks to the team at Eight Little Pages bringing it to life. I am grateful to James Essinger, for his support when I first completed the book. Thank you also to Thea Anderson for a very last minute read through.

I am privileged to have an amazing family. Thank you to my mum for teaching me to chase my dreams and to Zack, Cara and Dad for listening when I needed to talk. I am grateful to my brilliant family in-law, especially Angela for being the first person to read (and proofread!) this book. Also, thank you to John, Laura, Richard and the littlies for keeping me grounded.

Thank you to everybody who has put up with me rambling on about 'my book' for the last eight years! In particular, Veronica who has been my go-to girl for writing chats. She has been my personal cheerleader and I hope one day to repay the favour. I don't know what I would have done without my 'boob group' throughout my journey; they never fail to inspire me. Thank you to 'snack club' for continued bookish enthusiasm and mum-life support. I am also ever grateful to my band mates for always believing in me and being a sounding board for my ideas. Thank you to my university friends for celebrating with me every step of the way.

Finally, thank you to my virtual friends in the YouTube community, for the supportive comments and 'thumbs up' on my videos and posts. I am grateful to you for sharing your experiences, which were particularly useful when I needed help with the publishing process.

Of course, this book simply wouldn't have happened without my supportive, patient husband and wonderfully inspiring children. So, Stuart, Fin, Mae and Zoe, thank you, now and always.

MILK

1

BREASTFEEDING AND ME

It feels like we can't go a day without the subject of breast-feeding being on the TV, on the radio or in the press. Infant feeding, by whatever means, seems so divisive, so inflammatory. Why?

Breastfeeding doesn't need to be particularly interesting or exceptional, and everyone's experience is unique. My own breastfeeding journey has featured mountainous highs and deepest lows and I am just one person. This inspired me to pick up my laptop and start noting down my thoughts about breastfeeding, my research into it, and my personal experiences, eventually culminating in this book. I wanted to find out more about breastfeeding, and understand it better.

I'm a happily married mother of three. I live in Kent (the 'Garden of England') with my little family and until recently, when I started to focus more on writing, I worked as a biology teacher in a secondary school.

I've always been a maternal person, and children featured in my plans for the future. I just assumed I would breastfeed them and didn't ever think that doing so would be a big deal. But after cracked nipples, poor support, self-doubt and a ton of pressure (some of it self-inflicted), I came to realise that there was a hidden side to breastfeeding that needed to be discussed more openly. Too many of my friends suffered similar stories. Breastfeeding isn't as straightforward as it may seem.

Most women I'd talked to about breastfeeding told me it was 'lovely', or words to that effect. Friends, family, and even the parenting books I'd read, gave it a glow as rosy as the cheeks of a well-breastfed baby. You gaze lovingly at your little offspring as you provide sustenance to them with your own being. Why had nobody told me breastfeeding can be difficult? Why was I completely unaware of the pressures placed on mothers that make this natural process challenging? Why was the answer to every problem encountered to 'give up' and begin formula feeding? We need to start being honest about what is going on and fight for the right to feed our children as biology intended.

Women seem to clearly remember what it was like for them feeding their babies, even if decades have passed. When you talk about breastfeeding to a group of women the experiences they share can be wonderful or they can be raw, but they're always important. As a society our stories of breastfeeding teach us much about how we see women and how we see ourselves.

I fell pregnant for the first time around November 2009 and our second child was weaned in July 2014. I breastfed them both and, in June 2017, I started all over again after the birth of our third child.

In writing this, I've changed the names of all but my husband and children to protect the identities of those involved. My choice to expose my personal life doesn't have to be theirs. I've recalled conversations as accurately as I can, but they may not be word for word accurate.

2

MAMMALS AND MAMMARIES

Becoming pregnant for the first time made me extremely aware of my biology. I became increasingly conscious that I am an animal, who gives birth just as animals do in the wild, and feeds my baby in the same way too. My body was doing its thing without technology or any other human advance. I am intrinsically an animal, or, more accurately, a mammal.

I am glad I'm not an elephant, although pregnancy often made me feel like one. An elephant carries its baby for over a year and a half before birth. If I was anticipating a gestation of that length I think my apprehension might outweigh my excitement. Mammals aren't the only group that carry and give birth to live babies, for example, some sharks do too. Equally, not all mammals give birth, some, like the primitive monotremes, platypuses and echidnas, lay eggs. Laying an egg holds some appeal for me; it seems like much less fuss than childbirth, although I suppose sitting on a nest would be pretty boring. Egg-laying, along with other amphibious characteristics in monotreme mammals, may have allowed them to survive competition with marsupials in the past, by being able to hide in water.[1] This may be why, while other mammals have live births, monotremes still lay eggs.

The point is, though, carrying and birthing a live baby doesn't make me a mammal. No; the main defining feature of a mammal is that it secretes milk that is used to feed its young. That's why we, and our other furry friends, are called mammals. Eighteenth-century Swedish scientist and taxonomist Carl Linnaeus, best known for his work categorising living things, named our group after our mammary glands, a structure that only half of us use, which shows how important he thought it was.[2] I agree; I see lactation as our link to our animal cousins and our intrinsic biology.

Seeing a cow feeding her young is a common sight and we know what her milk is likely to look and taste like. We are familiar with how it's produced. But each mammal has its peculiarities when it comes to feeding their babies. For example, monotreme mammals don't even have nipples. Instead, milk is secreted on to the mother's skin from two mammary patches for her little nursling to lick from her fur.[3(pp18-20)]

Marsupial mammals also have their own idiosyncrasies. They don't have very long pregnancies.[4] Since they don't have placentas their ability to nourish their developing baby is limited. Instead, the baby is born at a very early stage and, almost miraculously, climbs straight to the mother's nipple inside her pouch. A newborn kangaroo, for example, looks like a red jelly bean and is about the same size. It has underdeveloped back legs, and so can only use its tiny front legs to climb up its mother's fur and down into her pouch, where it attaches itself (continuously at this stage) to one of her four nipples.[5] The mother's body then ejects milk into her baby's mouth.[4] The constantly changing milk in the pouch provides the nourishment mammals with placentas provide in the womb.[3(p36)] Once the baby is big enough it can let go of the nipple and eventually pop in and out of its mother's pouch and feed at will. By this point, the next tiny joey is already fastened to one of her other nipples.[7]

Placental mammals, such as us, are a varied bunch when it comes to lactation. Bats can feed upside down and whilst flying.[6] Cows, goats and sheep are farmed for their milk for another species (humans) to use. Hooded seals feed their young for just four days on the Arctic ice with the fattiest milk there is – 61% fat![7] Bears breastfeed their cubs whilst hibernating.[8] We all do it in our own way.

A blue whale, the largest mammal, has to coordinate feeding with diving. In order to remain streamlined, whales' nipples are hidden in skin folds near their tails.[9] Newborn blue whales drink enormous quantities of thick, fatty milk to help them grow quickly to an immense size.[10] Whales are born tail first and then rushed up to the surface to take their first lungful of air, breathing being a fairly important priority.[11] Nursing can then take place with the baby whale holding its breath underwater, the milk being forcibly ejected into the baby's mouth.[12] Human babies can breathe and breastfeed simultaneously,[13] but obviously living underwater makes this tricky for a whale.

Primates, such as ourselves and our ape cousins, provide our babies with comparatively dilute milk.[14] Humans, in particular, are born in a relatively primitive state due to the physical constraints of carrying and birthing a human infant to a comparative level of mental and physical development.[14] We primates also tend to feed our babies frequently; carrying them around with us.[14] We cannot leave our underdeveloped babies to fend for themselves; they could hardly run from a wolf or follow us to gather food. There is no need for energy rich milk that keeps a baby going for a long time while its parent is away; our babies are born snackers. We also tend to breastfeed for a number of years, since our babies spend a long time being babies compared to other species, to give our brains enough time to develop.

Humans, typically, have two nipples (as do other primates, goats, horses and guinea pigs). Other mammals have varying numbers of nipples; it generally depends on how many babies they usually have.[15] Nipples are ordinarily found in pairs down the 'milk lines',[16] although my dog, Dolly, weirdly has an odd number; nine to be exact. Most male mammals also have nipples and a couple can lactate (in extreme circumstances, even human males).[17]

It's hard to be sure how mammary glands evolved since nipples and glands don't preserve well as fossils.[18] Scientists, instead, have to look at living species and figure it out from there. It's generally thought that mammary glands evolved from sweat glands over 160 million years ago.[18] Milk was probably first used to keep eggs moist or, perhaps, to pass on immunity to young.[18] Over time the benefit of providing food for babies without having to go and find it for them – leaving the baby in peril – led to the evolution of breastfeeding.[14]

Providing milk from mammary glands creates a bond between mammal mothers and their babies that isn't available to non-mammals. Other creatures fend for their young in other ways. Many never even meet their babies; instead these offspring have to fend for themselves nutritionally from day one. The sea is full of planktonic babies looking out for themselves. Some creatures, such as birds, will eat food and then regurgitate it for their babies in a manageable form. Some creatures make special nutritional substances, such as bees and their honey. I like that we mammals care for our young in the physical way that we do. We give birth and we create sustenance with our own bodies. It has to be better than throwing up your food into your baby's mouth.

Breastfeeding is an essential part of our mammalian evolution and our reproductive biology. Women's bodies prepare for breastfeeding during puberty. Every menstrual cycle our breasts begin the journey to lactation, only continuing to develop if we conceive, otherwise returning to their resting state. Breastfeeding is a part of who we are.

3

LIFE BEFORE BABIES

I found giving birth incredible, revolutionary. At times I found motherhood overwhelming; sometimes wonderful and, at others, astoundingly hard. Without a network around me to pass on their experience and knowledge I don't know how I would have coped. Some people don't have information and support within easy reach and I can only imagine how hard that must be. I think it's even more essential to have this help when you are breastfeeding.

For something that is 'natural' for our bodies to do, breastfeeding is surprisingly difficult (or so I found). I assumed I would do it and it would be straightforward. I attended the classes and read the books. I imagined that with it being a biological process, which untold generations of women – and before them even more numerous generations of early humanoid mothers – had undertaken, it couldn't be complicated. I was wrong. Breastfeeding is amazing, beautiful, fascinating, emotional, challenging, and personal. I was about to go on a journey that would include downs as well as ups.

I knew few women who had successfully breastfed. My mother and mother-in-law had breastfed for short periods, but could remember little. I had one friend who had breast-fed a baby (others had formula-fed) but she was abroad for the most difficult first few months of motherhood so our exchanges were by email alone. Where I live, there is a breastfeeding support group, and it's a wonderful, warm-hearted collection of people. However, I can be shy and find it hard sometimes to strike up a conversation with a stranger. It was a while before I was confident enough to benefit from their knowledge. Nonetheless, I gradually met mothers with a variety of stories, and hearing another woman's experience was invaluable to me.

I think the place to start my tale is long before becoming pregnant. I'd like to start where I think my journey into breastfeeding began, when my breasts first showed themselves – puberty.

I can remember the early stages of my breasts developing, at around age nine. I felt both embarrassment and fascination that something was changing, forever. I was so excited when I got my first, cheap, AA cotton bra from the super-market. I felt like such a grown-up woman. I had to have a bra, not for support, but because the school shirts we wore were almost see-through and left nothing to the imagination. I have never understood why school shirts are made of the thinnest possible material. For the developing girl this was terrifying.

Once I was allowed to wear bras and crop tops I loved having pretty ones. I can clearly remember one cream satin crop top and shorts set I adored. It was so pretty and (I thought) sophisticated. Now, I am sure it would look childish, but back then it made me feel like a woman. Of course, even bras showed through our translucent school shirts, so as soon as you bought one you got a new barrage of comments and spent your days trying to stop boys from pinging your bra straps. You couldn't win either way. From the outset my breasts were a source of embarrassment to me, something that should be hidden, that made boys go into teasing mode and girls giggle.

I remember vividly the itchy feeling whilst my breasts expanded to their final size. It was maddening since it occurred at the worst times; in the middle of classes, in front of my friends' dads, at church...anywhere. I would have to either put up with it, or find a surreptitious way of scratching that nobody would see. I remember one of those awful 'puberty' lessons at school when the teacher told us about having to secretly scratch with your elbows while distracting from what you are doing by gesticulating with your hands. The idea stuck with me (probably because the lesson was so cringe-worthy) and so when my time came I gave it a go. It was a method I employed many times, probably causing me to look quite mad with my wildly flapping arms.

I felt I was becoming a woman, and truly I was, for what could be more symbolic of womanhood than your body preparing, visibly, to feed your future children. Bust size, in fact, has no bearing on the ability to breastfeed or the quantity of milk produced.[1] Women with the tiniest bosom are equal to those who are enormously endowed. I always felt fortunate in that I was somewhere in the middle.

Of course, puberty also resulted in all the other awkward changes that prepare you for childbearing later in life. I have broad hips (which I hated at the time), but my mum kept telling me I would appreciate them one day. I used to imagine being in labour next to a slim-hipped woman and saying, 'So who has the best shape now?'

It was fashionable to be tall and willowy back then, in the era of the 'waif', (and probably always will be). Girls with that physique seemed to me to symbolise what it meant to be cool. These girls also seemed to have the nicest and most expensive clothes, the right haircuts, and the best-looking boyfriends. I, however, always got it utterly wrong somehow. I was off to a bad start as I was short and curvy. My 'Rachel' haircut (from *Friends*) looked like a haystack due to my frizzy hair. I couldn't afford the Kickers school shoes, Adidas trousers or Nike trainers that everybody else wore. I started each new school year feeling sure I had got it right *this* time and would be brimming with confidence as I walked through the school gates with my new uniform, haircut, and make-up. But, every time, it was quickly clear that I was wrong and those tall, slim girls were right yet again.

To give an example, when I was about twelve, one of the cool girls had a lever arch folder covered in black and white fake fur, patterned like a Friesian cow. I thought it was super-cool, creative, tactile and original. Now, I was one of a handful of children at my school that had, for unknown reasons, purchased briefcases. I blame my mother for buying it; she claims I insisted I wanted one. I had already been teased about the fact that, as a twelve-year-old girl, I had a briefcase. I decided to take action. I was sure I could turn the situation around by borrowing this other girl's idea of style. I bought masses of leopard print fake fur and covered my briefcase in it. That would do the trick. I would now be the coolest girl in the school surely? I was going to be a trendsetter...no, *the* trendsetter.

In fact, my leopard print briefcase was not the amazing accessory I hoped for. The boys pretended it was attacking them and the girls raised their beautiful, plucked eyebrows and sniggered. I still can't bear leopard print materials.

On top of the jealousy I felt, these cool girls generally gave me a hard time at school which fuelled my hatred at the time. I must say that I have now largely got over my feelings towards tall, slim girls, although I do have the occasional unfortunate flashback of jealousy when I wish my legs were that little bit longer or my hips a fraction slimmer.

As my hips broadened a network of bright red lines webbed my thighs. At the tender age of about eleven I had never seen such a thing before. I had no idea what was wrong with me; it looked like some kind of alien disease. Rather than asking (and this was before internet search engines were commonplace) I tried to pretend it wasn't happening. This avoidance of help has become something of a pattern. At the time, I used to swim each weekend and when out of the pool I would spread my fingers wide, holding my hands against the raw marks, praying nobody would see them. I forget when I found out they were stretch marks, and common, but I learned to live with them once they had faded to a silvery white.

Of course, there was also the whole debacle of periods. It was the hot topic at school for a while. We had talks on what to expect and what to do. For some reason, one of the visiting teachers delivering these talks felt that a good demonstration of our future was sticking a sanitary towel to a girl's hand and making her wave. Is this normal? Perhaps it was to demonstrate flexibility or adhesiveness? We had boys' talks and girls' talks, and then, when we were a little older, we were led, sniggering, into the assembly hall to have a joint talk. There was a phase of boys rifling through girls' rucksacks to find the free sanitary towel samples we had squirrelled away. There was so much fascination; who had 'started', who hadn't? I was one of the early ones, but where, for some girls, it was a badge of honour they talked about persistently, I was inordinately embarrassed by the whole ordeal.

I emerged from puberty having been spared too much drama from my fluctuating hormones. I moved from middle school to upper school at the age of thirteen and started my new life, where not everybody remembered my briefcase.

At fourteen, once I was through the worst horrors of puberty, I met my husband-to-be, Stuart, at school. Our paths crossed when we both took part in the school production of *Little Shop of Horrors*. We were both in the chorus and would chat backstage while we waited for our sections of the show. His older sister, Laura, played Mrs Mushnik (the gender of the part having been changed because she was perfect in the role), but I was a little too much in awe of her to say anything but an occasional hello.

I didn't know back then that I would eventually marry Stuart. As in all good teenage romances we spent a few months insulting each other, before he summoned up the courage to ask me out. For instance, he would make jokes about my frizzy hair, while I would poke fun at him bringing little sachets of ketchup to have with his sandwiches at lunchtime. Thinking back, it was hard to figure out who was in love with you and who loathed you given that the signs were identical. In fact, if a boy spoke to you kindly (or at all) it probably showed ambivalence. Stuart was tall, with dark, curly hair and green eyes. I didn't especially fancy him in the beginning, it wasn't love at first sight, but I hung out with him in a hopeful sort of way.

Stuart had his uses. You see, I fancied his friend, Chris. So, I would hang around with them and try to give personal details to Stuart in the hope Chris would overhear and contact me. One day, I had given Stuart my email address (loudly, so Chris would hear) and the next thing I had an email asking me to come to his house for a double date with Laura and her then boyfriend, Gary. Well, I was not exactly inundated with invitations. I was pretty much bottom of the social heap.

At our school there were several social groups. The tall, skinny, cool girls already mentioned were at the top. The cool boys were generally sporty types, usually into football or rugby, and tall, strong and swoon-worthy. Next rung down you had the musical group. Their band T-shirts were clearly visible under their shirts and they were always on about 'Battle of the Bands' at the local under-sixteen's nightclub. Attached to them was the subgroup of musicians Stuart was in. They were generally liked by everyone and were sufficiently cool to get by. They played instruments and were in all the school productions and concerts and, on occasion, some great bands. But, I think their coolness came mostly through being allowed out of classes for music lessons.

Then there was my group. We were the best group I felt, because we were all ourselves, fiercely so. That was what held us together; we were against the world. But we were very uncool. To be seen with us was a social mistake. You did not hang out with the girl who had once had a leopard skin briefcase (and who now had a silver anorak and, in act of rebellion against the school uniform, wore an ankle length school skirt). Being asked out by someone from a higher social standing, i.e. Stuart, I couldn't help but be flattered. This didn't happen to the likes of me. He was also a really nice guy. So, I agreed.

4

MILK

We are used to pulling a bottle of milk from the fridge and it tasting or looking a certain way. But humans aren't cows and our milk is designed for human babies. The first milk produced by a mother is called colostrum. It is thick and yellow and so is often nicknamed 'liquid gold'. Sometimes, it appears to be clear though the colour varies. Either way, it contains nutrients that are extremely concentrated. A newborn baby's stomach is only about the size of a cherry and so the teaspoonful of milk that a baby can fit in there has to contain everything it needs.[1(p71)] Colostrum is also high in antibodies and other immune factors to help protect the baby while its immune system is getting started.[2(p45)]

When a baby breastfeeds for the first time it takes in microbes from its mother's skin.[3] The baby will already have managed to pick some up during birth as well.[4] Colostrum contains sugars called 'oligosaccharides' that feed those microbes.[3(p68)] It's pretty mind-blowing that milk feeds up babies' gut bacteria too! Also, contrary to popular belief, colostrum and breast milk aren't sterile.[4] Milk contains specific bacteria that the baby needs at a particular time.[5]

Around three or four days after birth a woman's milk starts to 'come in'. This is when colostrum noticeably turns to mature milk. Mothers might notice their breasts are heavier and their milk changes colour to the more familiar white. Mature breast milk contains all the food groups as you would expect: vitamins, minerals, proteins, fats and carbohydrates (mostly lactose).[6] Like colostrum it contains immune factors[7] and 'friendly' bacteria,[3(p68)] but in different quantities.

The make-up of milk changes all the time. During a feed the fat content will increase,[7] perhaps turning more from a drink to a meal. Equally, over a day milk will change; it has even been found that breast milk at night contains sleep-inducing hormones![8] Milk for an older child will be different to that for a younger one.[1(pp29-30)] Milk for a boy can be different to that for a girl.[9] Milk will even be a different consistency depending on the weather; being more thirst quenching if it's hot.[10] If two different children are feeding at the same time each breast can also be a different temperature so the child is not too warm or cold.[11] It is perfectly tailor-made and very clever.

Human milk is thinner than the cow's milk that a lot of us will be more familiar with, but it's sweeter.[7] I think it tastes like sweet, skimmed cow's milk. I have tried it; curiosity got the better of me. I know some people find the idea of drinking human milk gross (although I suppose trying your own is not quite as weird...or is it?). It's funny that we are more familiar with another species' milk than our own, to the point where some people are squeamish about human milk but will think nothing of drinking pint after pint of cow's milk. Anyway, since human milk is different in composition to other mammals' milk it isn't a good idea to simply give a baby milk from another species. Currently formula milk is used as a substitute and that is derived from cow's milk. However, it's designed to have similarities to human milk so that it's safe for human babies.

Natural production of breast milk is controlled by a delicate balance of hormones. The hormone 'prolactin' makes the breasts produce milk.[12] The more you feed, the more prolactin you produce, and then the more milk you produce.[2(p10)] It's a supply and demand system. The more you breastfeed; the more milk you make. If you feed less, your body makes less. One of the other main hormones involved is oxytocin, the love hormone (and my favourite hormone, if I can have a favourite). This is the same hormone you release when you stroke an animal, hug a friend, or have an orgasm.[13] It shouldn't be a surprise that breastfeeding can give a feeling of love, well-being, bonding...however you like to describe it. Oxytocin makes tiny muscles in the lobules of breast tissue contract to eject milk.[1(p24)] It's also the hormone responsible for ramping up labour and causing the uterus to contract,[14] which is something I am, perhaps, a little less keen on.

But oxytocin isn't just something you make when you breastfeed, it's something you make when you are in love.

5

LOVE STORY

It was to be my first proper date, a double date at that! I had wondered if I would ever date anyone, given my weirdness. But here I was being invited into the home of someone more cool than me, someone nice, and funny. I was incredulous that *he* had asked *me* out, not the other way around. I also had a bit of a crush on Stuart's beautiful, flame-haired sister, in a sort of 'I want to be you' way. Laura had once said my hairclip was pretty and I had been so thrilled I wore it for about a year. So, I was nervous on both fronts. I didn't know how to dress (fortunately, I don't remember whatever weird ensemble I chose) and I was worried about how to act.

My mum drove me the three miles to Stuart's house. I was paranoid I had noted down the wrong address, but when I rang the doorbell Stuart answered, smiling. His parents were out since Laura (just over a year older than us at sixteen) was deemed old enough and sensible enough to take responsibility for us.

Laura had cooked, I forget exactly what. We sat around the table in the kitchen (their home being sufficiently large to have a table in the kitchen as well as a separate dining room – a rarity in Britain), which made it more informal. We were each handed a napkin with a specially chosen napkin ring (mine was a pewter duck, I think) and I started to worry about table etiquette and the like. Of course, I'd used a napkin before, just not at home. It was a sign they were more posh than me and I was worried that I would show myself up.

However, I was treated like an old friend by Stuart, Laura and Gary. I felt liked, which was a rare enough event where my peers were concerned. I started to relax as I realised I did fit in with this little social group. Whenever I told an anecdote Laura would put down her cutlery and listen intently, like I was absolutely fascinating. It seemed such a classy thing to do for a guest, to make them feel that interesting, and had the effect of making me feel genuinely liked.

When we finished eating Stuart and I went up to his room. He had a small twelve-inch television and a VCR and had rented the film *Face Off*, which, it transpired, we both thought was lame. We sat on his bed making jokes about the film until, halfway through, I heard the doorbell ring downstairs. Laura announced that my mum had come to pick me up and so, my first date was at an end.

I left with a smile on my face. It turned out that the boy who hadn't caught my attention at school was actually a lovely, likeable, attractive, genuine and honest guy. He made me feel good about myself. The next Monday at school we were holding hands in the playground. My friend

Veronica asked, 'Are you two going out then?' We looked at each other sheepishly and seemed to wordlessly agree.

'Yes,' we replied. Veronica still credits herself for our relationship because she was the one who formalised it.

We were immediately inseparable at that tender age of fourteen and quickly became one of those couples at school who are *always* together. We kissed passionately at the bus stop before he left to go home as if we were to be parted forever. We spent our lunchtimes locked in each other's arms. We argued fiercely in the middle of the playground as my fiery, hormone-fuelled temper flared up at the tiniest provocation.

I can remember us having an understanding, even early on, that we both intended to have children one day and I have some recollection of discussing with Stuart how many we would have and what we would call them. Not that we had any intention of conceiving back then, rather, we simply made it clear that we both wanted children 'when we grew up' as we both felt a long, meaningful, relationship with somebody that didn't want children was pointless. How sensible at such a young age!

We went to different universities, but managed to stay together. I studied Marine Biology at Plymouth. This degree path had become inevitable after my first SCUBA dive at age thirteen. My dad served fifteen years in the Royal Navy and, for some of that time, had been a ship's diver. My parents split up when I was five and, when I was nine, my dad moved to Saudi Arabia. He rediscovered diving in the Red Sea and quickly got through the training to become an instructor. So, when I visited him, he was desperate for me to try it. I reluctantly agreed; I was a bit scared in case I drowned or got eaten by a shark.

My first sea dives took place in Jeddah, on the Red Sea. The underwater world there is teeming with the most vividly coloured life and I quickly forgot any anxiety; I was instantly hooked. There were fish of every colour and size swimming close enough to touch. Coral formed the hills and trees of this land, with white sand valleys running in between.

On my third dive my dad took me to visit a section of reef that had been bulldozed to build an artificial beach. The jewelled tones gave way to grey, barren rock. A handful of fish swam slowly, as though lost, through the piles of white coral skeletons. My eyes filled with tears. My life changed right then. The marine world became my passion.

It was easy to choose what I wanted to study for three years. By then I had amassed around sixty dives, all in the Red Sea, and I was eager to learn about everything I'd seen there as well as take a peek at the waters around the British Isles. Stuart, on the other hand, had decided to study Chemistry in Canterbury, some 270 miles away.

I loved living in the south-west of England. I had lived most of my life as far as it was possible to get from the sea but now it was within walking distance. I would sit on Plymouth Hoe by the red and white striped lighthouse looking out at the navy ships dotted around Drake's Island that occupied the centre of the bay. Whenever I could, I would jump on my bike and cycle through the most beautiful woodlands into Dartmoor and sit under a tree by the River Plym to read my course books. My friends and I would grab our dive kits, jump in the car and drive to so many beautiful coastal villages where we explored the undersea world. Cawsand Bay in Cornwall was one of our favourite haunts and we desperately (unsuccessfully) searched for seahorses among the seagrass there. I was at my happiest hovering weightless over a six foot high kelp forest watching the creatures that called it home. As my mum once said to me, 'Who knew there were so many fish in the sea?'

I sat enraptured in lectures about things that I was hugely passionate about, and totally bored in others I didn't understand. I read and wrote late into the night and slept late into the day. I spent a summer in Greece volunteering for a turtle conservation charity, ensuring the tiny babies made it safely into the sea from their beach nests. I went clubbing and drank far too much, far too often, knowing I wouldn't be this young and free again. I laughed and lived as much as I could and I didn't regret a moment.

For Stuart things hadn't worked out at university. He hadn't found his degree interesting and hadn't enjoyed student life. He decided to work until he chose what path to follow instead. He had a job in Canterbury, near to his family. I was still studying. Jobs in the south-west are hard to come by and neither of us was ready for him to relocate so we lived apart.

Midway through my degree I spent a summer with Stuart as an experiment to see if we could live together. We were concerned the long-distance relationship might be an illusion and once we were together all the time we would drive each other crazy. During this long summer we booked a week's holiday together, our first since leaving home. We chose the Czech capital Prague because it was purportedly cheap and beautiful, a perfect combination. Neither of us had any money for an extravagant trip but we still wanted to do something romantic together since we spent such precious little time with one another.

I had my suspicions about Stuart's intentions. His sister had talked a lot about jewellery, asking me whether I preferred gold or silver, for example. Stuart seemed preoccupied. So, in order to prevent getting a surprise, and to be thoroughly in control of the situation as I liked to be, I searched our room and our luggage. No ring. I could relax; there were no surprises in store. Except, having kept the ring at his sister's house, the sneak had snuck it into his pocket. He must have been thankful that he didn't have to empty his pockets at airport security.

Having arrived in Prague and checked into our hotel we went for a walk. With me sitting on a bench atop a hill Stuart got down on one knee and asked me the question I had been so sure he wouldn't be asking during that holiday.

'Will you marry me?' he asked, producing the ring from his pocket where it had been hidden.

'Yes,' I answered immediately. I had envisioned this moment for as long as I had known what a proposal was. Here was my childhood sweetheart, knelt before me in a stunning European city, asking little old me to marry him. I didn't need to think about my reply. After all, I had imagined this moment a thousand times before. As my heart raced he slipped the trilogy diamond ring on to my finger.

On closer inspection, once the excitement had died away a little, it wasn't quite the idyllic spot Stuart had hoped for. It was covered in graffiti and full of dog muck. It didn't matter. He could have asked anywhere and I would have given the same answer. Plus, Stuart had been forced to propose as soon as possible because he knew I was suspicious and on high alert for any signs that it was imminent. We were also staying in a tiny hotel room with limited hiding places and so the ring wasn't going to stay secret for much longer.

I returned to Plymouth as one of the few students sporting a rock on their finger. My final year vanished before I knew it, heralding the start of real grown-up life. I would have to seek gainful employment for a start. But there was also the issue of my personal life. We still lived in opposite corners of the country. Although Britain is a relatively small island, that is still fairly prohibitive of a meaningful relationship in the long term.

I adored Devon and Cornwall and the glorious, dramatic rocky beaches. I knew the best dive spots and knew where to find particular creatures as I had dived along much of the local coast. I loved the friendliness of the local people and I hoped to pick up their beautiful accent. It didn't even matter that it rained a lot of the time. No other part of the country held the same enchantment, and it still doesn't. It will always be my spiritual home.

But the romance of a place isn't as important as the practicalities of life, unfortunately. A place will still be there (although perhaps changed) when you visit, or return. A marriage is less likely to be. Stuart also wanted to stay where he was. Our families were in the south-east, as were potential jobs. Although my heart yearned to stay in the west, sense told me to move. So, we settled in Kent, which is beautiful enough to quell my thoughts of the south-west and close enough to our families that we could be a part of life. Most importantly, we were together.

We had a quintessentially English country wedding. I had flowers and berries in my hair and Stuart wore a morning suit. The Norman country church (which I had frequented for most of my life pre-university) made a beautiful setting for the ceremony. The reception was in a local village hall with a game of cricket taking place on the lawn. We drank Pimm's and danced to a jazz band in which the best man played trombone.

For a long time afterwards we struggled financially as we tried to find careers that we could settle into for an extended period so we could get a mortgage and then, hopefully, have children. One or other of us would always be training. Stuart had, by then, found a college course that suited him in electronics and, as soon as he finished, I started training as a teacher. We supported each other financially through this time; so our situation wasn't sufficiently stable for a while to seriously consider starting a family.

I think people had expected babies to come sooner. I suppose when you get married people assume that is the next step. We weren't ready for that yet. By the time we did get around to having children I was sick of people asking when we were going to have them or alluding to it. I really wanted children, I always had. Other people talking about it felt like rubbing my nose in the fact that I was *still* childless. It got to the point where it felt like a huge intrusion into my privacy, like asking about our sex life. I know it was simply other people's excitement, but that didn't stop the irritation. As time went on pressure seemed to mount.

Motherhood was something I craved; I counted down the days until a time when we would be secure enough financially and emotionally to consider parenthood. As a little girl I had played endlessly with baby dolls, cuddling them and putting them to bed under any blanket I could find. When I was a teenager I was the primary babysitter in my road. By the time I was in my twenties there was a nagging hole in my life and I had to do something about it.

We worked hard to reach a point where pregnancy could be a consideration. We ensured we had good jobs. I finally qualified and was working as a biology teacher in a grammar school. Stuart got a great job as an electronics technician with a railway transport company. We then waited until we were lucky enough to buy a home, ready to fill with babies. At twenty-five years old, having been married for three years and together for eleven, we were *finally* ready to start a family. It felt weird, to be at that point where our lives were to make a complete change. But, it had been a milestone for so long that the excitement far outweighed the worry.

I had spent hour upon hour reading up on the internet about conception, long before it was a possibility for us. There was little I didn't know. As the time drew near I forced zinc and vitamin C down Stuart's throat (which I'd heard boosts fertility)[1] and took folic acid myself (this reduces the risk of neural tube defects such as spina bifida).[2] Once I had calculated the earliest possible time having a child would be feasible (to ensure optimal maternity leave at work) I demanded we try immediately, to Stuart's delight.

About a fortnight after we started trying for a baby I went away with my three closest girlfriends, one of whom was pregnant with her second child. We were having a weekend in a fancy hotel that had a pool, saunas and steam-rooms. I was gutted I wouldn't be able to use them, since they supposedly aren't advisable in pregnancy.[3] After staying out of the Jacuzzi and generally acting a bit weird I came clean to my friends that I was trying for a baby. I would have had to tell them anyway as I couldn't drink alcohol and that may have been a give-away as I was generally one to have a glass (or three) of wine.

They were excited and convinced I must already be pregnant. One friend announced she had known subliminally that I was trying for a baby. It was nice that others had such confidence in my fertility. It was also a relief to be able to talk to somebody about it (Stuart and I were keeping things quiet from the family to reduce the pressure). We spent the weekend discussing babies and my pregnant friend made it her mission to tell me everything she could about her first pregnancy and birth so I was prepared. Unfortunately, breastfeeding never came into the conversation.

I expected months of uncertainty and complications, especially since issues surrounding conception are often played out on television and have also, unfortunately, been experienced by some of my friends. But it turned out the girls were right; I was already pregnant during that weekend away.

I knew I was pregnant. I don't know how, but I knew. I quickly became increasingly emotional, coming home from work in tears and generally being difficult to live with as my hormones fluctuated. I had already stocked up on pregnancy tests the second we started trying for a baby. So, a few days before my period was meant to start I decided that, although it was early, I was going to try a test. I knew they don't generally work until you have missed your period (unless you have those super fancy ones), but I couldn't handle the suspense any longer.

It was the first time I had ever taken a pregnancy test. I carefully read the instructions to make sure I knew how to go about it and conveniently ignored the bits about it not working until you had missed a period. Feeling nervous, I urinated on the stick. I then waited the allotted time, anxiously anticipating the little blue line. There was nothing. Although I knew it wasn't a 'no' as such, just a 'too early', I was crestfallen.

A week later I did another test as my period still hadn't shown up. I can be late, especially if I'm under any kind of stress (such as trying to conceive) so that wasn't conclusive evidence. After weeing on the stick I decided to while away the time so my thundering heart didn't arrest. I distracted myself with Facebook and tried not to look obsessively at the little window on the test.

After a minute, I glanced down and thought I saw a pale line but convinced myself I was seeing things so looked away quickly. Besides, the two minutes weren't up. I was so excited I couldn't help sneaking another glance. It was still there. I picked the test up and examined it more closely. I put it down and went back on Facebook, wondering if maybe, when the two minutes were up, the line would disappear. Perhaps it appears and then vanishes again? I looked once more, convinced I would find it was a figment of my imagination. After some time, Stuart called up the stairs, eagerly awaiting the verdict himself. When I didn't respond he came upstairs and I wordlessly showed him the test. He could see the line too. I hadn't imagined it, I really was pregnant.

I was reeling. Discovering I was pregnant sent me into shock. Although, of course, I was delighted, I hadn't expected it to be so easy. We sat eating dinner in near silence, me shaking and Stuart smiling, absorbing the news. It was the weirdest evening, with everything as it normally was except for one huge new fact, a tiny wonder in my womb that was going to change everything.

6

THE HISTORY OF BREASTFEEDING

In that moment I joined the ranks of billions of women who had reproduced. I felt linked by this shared experience through the whole of human history. I was on my way to becoming a mother, the creator of a generation.

I was also on my way to breastfeeding. The history of breastfeeding had an impact on my experience as it will for anyone. If we know what has gone before it helps us to understand why things are the way they are and to cope with the frustrations we are dealt with.

Prehistoric women would have breastfed their babies. There wouldn't have been an alternative choice; it was simply how a baby was fed. Tribal women continue to do this and we can look at their cultures to get an idea of how humans would have breastfed in pre-agricultural times.

The !Kung tribe (the ! in their name is a clicking sound) of the Kalahari Desert is often used as an example.[1(p138)] They are a hunter-gatherer society that also practice small scale farming.[2(p39)] !Kung mothers carry their babies naked in a sling while they forage, allowing the baby to breastfeed when they wish, with no thought as to whether it's too often or for too long.[2(p39)] During the night they both lie on the mother's cloak and the baby continues to breastfeed at will.[2(p39)] !Kung babies typically breastfeed for three and a half years, which helps the mother to space out pregnancies due to the contraceptive effect of frequent breastfeeding.[3]

As society changes, so does the role of women and the culture of breastfeeding. Women in Western society have become less likely to live in the social groups that are more natural for humans, meaning we can't help each other with daily tasks or with baby care. This has made breastfeeding harder because it increases the burden on the mother who cannot share her load when she needs to feed her baby.

Women who need to work cannot always do so and breastfeed their babies. In some instances, in the past, women may have been able to work with their babies, carrying them like the !Kung. But often a working mother has to be separated from her child meaning it must be fed a different way.

There has always been a place for an alternative to breastfeeding, whether because a mother is working, she cannot breastfeed for physiological reasons, she is ill, or because she has died. Formula milk only became available in the late nineteenth century and, of course, was only safe when the milk from which it was sourced was clean.[4] Prior to this, a wet nurse would usually be found to feed the birth mother's children. This practice is less commonplace now but it raises complex issues about relationships and biology nonetheless.

Over time, feeding another woman's baby became something you could get paid for (or pay someone to do) and it came to be called 'wet nursing'. It began to turn from something that occurred when it was needed to something you could choose to do for convenience or fashion.[4] It is among the oldest professions, having its roots around 2000 BC.[4]

Wet nursing is an age-long tradition that spans cultures, with King Tutankhamen having built an amazing tomb for his wet nurse, Maia.[2(p65)] Examples are documented in Ancient Rome and in the Bible.[4] When a wet nurse was sought by the Pharaoh's daughter for the baby Moses, his biological mother was secured for the task.[5] In Ancient Rome unwanted, discarded female babies would be bought to be slaves and nursed by slave wet nurses.[4] There was little alternative until formula came about. Women nursed each other's babies as a favour or as paid work.

Of course, wet nursing is still breastfeeding and provides human milk for a human baby. However, the milk of another woman will never be as tailor-made for your baby as your own, especially in terms of passing on immunity.[6] A wet nurse might not have been exposed to the same illnesses or live in the same area as the birth mother, so her milk will not contain the perfect antibodies.

For the most part, wet nurses would have been employed by rich families. The only exception was when a mother died or abandoned her baby. Poor people simply couldn't afford wet nurses. In sixteenth-century Europe, noble women would be expected to be sexually attractive and able to have a baby at a moment's notice.[7] Breastfeeding doesn't sit well with that image. Virginal, firm breasts were the ideal to aspire to.[6] Breastfeeding also has a contraceptive effect and so it would reduce the rate that a woman could produce heirs.[1(p182)] Rich women (or often their husbands) would hire wet nurses to feed their babies[1(p187)] so they could be fashionably sexy and produce as many heirs as possible.

Wet nursing was so common by the seventeenth and eighteenth centuries in Western Europe that only the very poorest women fed their own babies.[2(p66)] It was so prevalent that even wet nurses hired cheaper wet nurses to feed their babies while they worked for richer employers.[2(p66)] Poor women may have informally fed each other's babies (for instance, sisters or friends might help each other out with feeding), but they couldn't afford to hire somebody to do it.

Wet nurses, all too often, gave poor care to the babies they were paid to breastfeed, so the mortality rate rose.[4] This was particularly the case when babies were sent away to a wet nurse rather than when one lived with the family. Wet nurses in the country often took on more babies than they could handle, so they wouldn't be able to care for them all well enough, and conditions were generally poor.[8] Wet nurses who lived with their employees might generally have cared better for the infants but would often be forced to give up their own children, at least for the duration of their employment.[1(p188)]

In France, death rates from neglect by wet nurses were particularly high and this led to a drive to encourage women to feed their own babies.[8] The French philosopher, Jean-Jacques Rousseau, in his famous book *Emile* described the perfect way to bring up a child, this boy called Emile. One of the important aspects was for him to have been breastfed by his own mother. He argued:

When mothers deign to nurse their own children, then there will be a reform in morals; natural feeling will revive in every heart; there will be no lack of citizens for the state; this first step by itself will restore mutual affection.[9]

This was around the time Carl Linnaeus named our group of animals 'mammals'. As well as being a biologist, Linnaeus was a doctor, known for being against the practice of wet nursing for medical and natural reasons.[8] Using the name 'mammal' perhaps also made a point by emphasising our most important feature.[8]

Wet nurses became less common in Europe after the eighteenth century due to efforts to discourage their use.[8] Richer women started feeding their own babies again.[6] The idea that breastfeeding was for poor women only started to change.[4] Interestingly, now we find ourselves in the opposite situation. It's more common for wealthy women to breastfeed in the Western world and so we're more likely to link poor women with formula feeding in our perceptions and prejudices.[2(pp286-287)]

In North America, seventeenth-century European settlers looked for wet nurses so they could carry on in the cultural tradition they were used to. They looked to the native populations because they were seen as lower status.[2(p67)] In the eighteenth century, black slaves in the South would wet nurse their white mistresses' babies, at the expense of their own children.[2(p67)]

In Muslim countries breastfeeding has enjoyed a more protected status. The Qu'ran specifies that babies should be breastfed for a protracted amount of time, for instance: *In travail upon travail did his mother bear him. And in years twain was his weaning.*[10] Therefore, if a mother can't feed her baby for any reason wet nursing would be the preferred alternative.[11] In Islam, a child that is wet nursed is regarded as a sibling to the wet nurse's own children and as such cannot marry them.[12]

The culture of wet nursing had a significant effect on breastfeeding wherever it occurred. Elsewhere, breastfeeding continued to be the primary form of infant feeding.[2(p75)] This just goes to show that cultural issues with breastfeeding are not a modern phenomenon. By the twentieth century wet nursing was largely replaced with the use of infant formula which has become far more prevalent than wet nursing ever was.

Until the invention of the bottle it was difficult to feed a baby any alternative to breast milk. Clay feeding vessels have been found that date from 2000 BC onwards.[4] Sadly, they were found in the graves of the babies that could have died as a result of their use. Other materials have been used, including hollow animal horns, wood and silver, typically featuring a spout for the baby to feed from.[4] Without the knowledge and materials of later years it was impossible to keep them clean and bacteria-free, contributing to many infant deaths.[4] In the nineteenth century the first glass bottles appeared.[4] These were much more successful and went on to be refined and adapted into the plastic designs with soft teats we see today.

In the sixteenth century there was a belief that wet nurses could pass on syphilis, which was at epidemic proportions at the time.[1(p177)] It's thought this may have been a part of the drive to find alternative foods for babies. Of course, people have tried to feed babies with other foods for all sorts of reasons; the most obvious alternative being animal milk.[4]

Before the advent of pasteurisation or the refrigerator, using milk was a risky business. Milk had to be drunk fresh. For instance, in French foundling hospitals of the 1700s goats would be kept for the infants to feed from directly, there is nothing fresher! It's reported that in Aix-en-Provence the goats would actually straddle the cots, which must have been quite a sight.[13] Milk would also be given in feeding vessels and, without modern preservation techniques, it's no great surprise that the use of animal milk was only really successful in colder climates, where it's less dangerous because microbes don't flourish so well.[2(p78)] Nonetheless, babies fed animal milks often died due to contamination.[4]

Historically, most people wouldn't have used animal milk at all, until it was introduced by Europeans, let alone give it to babies.[7] In fact, most human adults lack the enzyme to digest cow's milk, we're only meant to drink milk from our own species.[1(p17)] A variety of animal milks have been used to feed babies, depending on the animals available. Babies have been fed with donkey milk, pig milk, horse milk...but, ultimately, the most popular has been cow's milk.[4]

Pap was another alternative, often used to supplement animal milk if babies failed to thrive.[4] Pap is a mixture of bread, water and milk. These mixtures too would quickly go off which, added to the poor nutritional value and the non-sterile feeding utensils, made them a deadly substance. In the Dublin Foundling Hospital in the eighteenth century almost every baby fed this way died.[1(p178)] This was repeated wherever pap was used.

Breast milk was a valuable substance. It has also been used medicinally, even for adults, with evidence for the practice dating back to the sixteenth century when it was used as a pain reliever.[7] It was sometimes used to treat blindness, hysteria and ear infections (I am sure with varying success).[7] Most likely, its use in eye treatments arose from women using breast milk to treat minor eye infections in babies.[7] This is something which still continues today due to the anti-infective properties of breast milk. I've tried it and it genuinely works. Breast milk was also used as an easily digested food for weak adults, such as those with consumption.[8] Research in the last twenty years has shown that a compound derived from breast milk even makes cancer cells 'commit suicide'.[14] As a result, some cancer patients have tried drinking breast milk as an alternative therapy, with some swearing it alleviated the symptoms.

However successful breast milk's healing powers have been for each illness, its use in this way shows how important it was (and is) culturally. It was a fount of life.

Elsewhere in the world substitutes for breast milk have been less rarely sought. In Japan, for example, if a mother didn't produce enough milk, medicines, prayer or wet nursing would be used (wet nursing was only used when it was really needed).[15] Babies were not fed to a set pattern, were kept skin-to-skin with the mother and weaned aged two or three.[15] Similarly to the West, once the bottle took over from wet nursing in the late nineteenth century this led to a rise in infant mortality.[15]

As already stated, breastfeeding is protected and promoted in Islam, so breastfeeding in the Middle East has been relatively unharmed. Wet nursing would be used, if necessary, as a preference to artificial means. Even Mohammed had two wet nurses. In Islam a wet nurse becomes a relative, a milk-mother.[12] This fact could even be used in negotiations in a similar way to the use of marriage for political means; a milk-kinship could be set-up.[12] Today, wet nursing continues to be common in some areas although, in others, formula feeding has taken over.[11]

In developing nations, breastfeeding rates are higher where there is less access to formula milk.[2(p51)] The practices of carrying babies and sleeping with them are also common in these cultures. Wherever communities haven't been disrupted by urbanisation, marketing and the like, breastfeeding is better preserved.

Generally, over the course of history, babies have struggled to survive without human milk, ideally from the natural mother. The last century has seen that change with the popularity of formula milk which is now largely safe. But, until then, breast milk was essential for survival. That still didn't mean breastfeeding was without obstacles.

Throughout history we have seen an impact from 'expert advice', both positive and negative. It doesn't take much of an internet search to see how much conflicting 'advice' there is even now.

Male 'experts' tried to reform breastfeeding; to professionalise and medicalise it. Advice for mothers began to appear in the sixteenth century from medical writers who promoted breastfeeding and linked it with good mothering.[7] This was to try and tackle the problems created by widespread, fashionable wet nursing amongst the rich. They recognised the infant period was an important and uncertain time and so advice began to be published on every aspect of baby care.[7] Through the seventeenth and eighteenth centuries, rich women could turn to these writings for advice on breastfeeding, or indeed any other aspect of baby care, as they re-learnt the art of breastfeeding which had been lost to their class.[7]

Traditionally, women would have given each other information about breastfeeding through experience sharing[8] and observation.[1(p45)] Poorer women would have carried on doing exactly that.[7] Richer women may have had no peers to turn to for these shared experiences because few of them had breastfed their babies. They had nowhere to turn but to 'experts'.

The advice was mixed. Doctors believed stress could affect milk, including childbirth. Some believed milk should be withheld until the woman stopped bleeding after childbirth, which can last as long as six weeks.[7] Without the baby suckling in that interim period, breast milk production would be threatened. Women who couldn't afford to employ wet nurses wouldn't have been able to follow this advice; they would have no choice but to breastfeed initially and so breastfeeding was unharmed.[7] Again, poorer women were more successful at breastfeeding during this period.

In time, medical experts realised early feeding was important and began to write about the merits of colostrum.[7] Its yellowish colour meant that, for centuries, it had been understood that colostrum was different from usual breast milk but its importance was not always recognised. For example, it was common practice in the eighteenth century for women to give alternative milks or secure a wet nurse until their milk 'came in' rather than to feed colostrum to their babies.[7] Tackling this wasn't only safer for babies (because they weren't being given contaminated foods and because they were getting an immunological hit from the colostrum) but also caused a rise in breastfeeding numbers because it helped women to get breastfeeding started.[7] Experts at this time also advocated feeding on demand; giving milk little and often as our species naturally does.[7]

William Cadogan, a well-known doctor of eighteenth-century Britain, was an ardent advocate of babies being breastfed by their own mothers, with no other food being given until it was time to wean on to solids.[1(p24)] This was wonderful advice in the wake of commonplace wet nursing. In that respect he single-handedly lowered the rate of infant mortality and made breastfeeding fashionable again. However, he also believed babies were dying from overfeeding (it was actually due to them eating contaminated foods) and so he advised only feeding a baby four times a day and discouraged feeding at night.[1(p24)] Anyone spending much time around a newborn would soon realise this is impossible without starving and distressing the baby. Still, Cadogan started the trend of following routine. Since milk production is governed by a 'supply and demand' system, the limiting of feeds through strict, regular routine has a significant impact on milk production. Proponents of routine have continued to this day and still it causes problems with breastfeeding.[16] His legacy has been mixed.

Breastfeeding was known to be hard work. Women who could afford wet nurses sometimes chose to employ one for convenience.[7] Also there were concerns over health. In a time without antibiotics, mastitis must have been terrifying. In some instances breastfeeding could scar, deform and even kill, if an infection could not be treated.[7] This would have been even more common in women who were badly informed and so prone to damaged nipples or blocked ducts. In the same way well-meaning relatives may pressure women to bottle-feed now, the pressure to get a wet nurse back then would have been similar.[7] You wouldn't want your loved ones to take those risks or to work that hard when they could pay someone else to do it.

Still, women who could breastfeed were respected and valued in a time when many rich women either could not, or would not, breastfeed. There was a contention between the importance of breastfeeding and the cultural issues that meant women struggled to do it. We still see the same now.

I was following in the footsteps of generations of women who had been influenced by prevailing cultural ideas about breastfeeding. I had so much to learn as I prepared for this baby. It wasn't going to be easy and, it seems, it never has been.

7

WAITING FOR BABY

I spent the next few weeks having to appear nonchalantly normal whilst I was actually feeling extremely nervous. I felt as though I was so bursting with the knowledge of my 'condition' that people must be able to read it on my face. I tried not to moon about, touching my, as yet, flat belly. I worried that I may suddenly develop Tourette's-like symptoms and have no control over the random, inappropriate shouting of 'I'm pregnant!' I tried to act normally, but nothing was normal, nothing at all.

The first symptom I suffered from was the emotional results of my raging hormones. I was tearful and quick to anger. It felt very similar to PMT. The horrible thing about hormonal rage is the knowing looks in people's eyes (sometimes those thoughts are put into words, hurtfully). I think an angry woman is assumed to be an irrational woman governed by the chemical messengers parading around in her bloodstream. However, sometimes I am angry because something has annoyed me. Sometimes, I am angry even when I am far from menstruating. Sometimes, I am angry *even though I am menstruating* and I am completely justified in that rage. Even when it seems I am irrational, being hormonal doesn't make my anger any less real. If nobody annoyed me then I wouldn't be angry. Therefore, there is justification since there is provocation, even if the end result may be a little excessive. My point is, women are allowed to be angry and their hormones ought to be disregarded.

The next early symptom was the ache in my poor, sore breasts and so my route to breastfeeding began in earnest. It hurt to walk, since the tiniest wobble of my flesh felt like bruising. I have run up and down stairs for as long as I can remember. My mum always said I sounded like a herd of elephants going up and down the stairs, being chased by our border collie nipping at my heels and barking. However, now, running *anywhere* was unthinkable. Instead, I had to walk carefully whilst holding my breasts still with my hands. It also hurt to lie in any position that resulted in their compression.

It even hurt to wear certain clothes. Underwired bras were torturous and so I was forced to buy fabric bras. They closely resembled my first training bras, but I was now a C cup, not AA. Since the early days of having breasts I have worn padded bras to give me a rounded shape and to avoid 'peanut smuggling', but now I was forced to wear lots of layers instead to hide the lack of support. Nonetheless, my unappealing new bras didn't hurt so I had to put up with the aesthetic issues. At night, I needed clothing that would stop any part of my breast getting caught under my arm and to minimise movement. So, I ended up buying sleep bras as well, like soft crop tops. Along with this, I was frantically worried about the possible sagging that pregnancy may cause, so any kind of opposition to gravity, even at night, seemed like an extremely good idea.

A pattern of bumps appeared around my nipples that didn't used to be there. These are 'Montgomery tubercles', glands that secrete oil so your nipples stay supple, which can be helpful for breastfeeding.[1] They're already there but often become more obvious once you are pregnant. This change was fairly insignificant to me. But next, my areolas darkened and appeared to get larger. I found this hard to handle. This was the only change in skin colour I experienced, I didn't get a *linea nigra* (a line from your belly button to your pubic hair), and I didn't get any discoloration on my face.[2] I didn't know if the colour change in my nipples was permanent or not (it turns out it wasn't entirely) but I liked the way I was; I didn't want change. It's funny the things that do, or don't, affect you. I had long accepted the inevitable big bump, the possible stretch marks, the huge boobs, but this one was new to me and I hadn't had a chance to come to terms with it.

I felt torn between excitement and horror concerning the changes to my body. I knew I was undergoing a metamorphosis that was unlikely to be entirely reversible and, quite frankly, it terrified me. I was proud of my body and had few hang-ups. I had come to like the way I looked and had finally learnt to appreciate what I had. Short and curvy I may always be, but I was also slim and had an 'hourglass' figure. I did karate and was fairly fit and strong; I looked after myself. I didn't want to go through that process of getting to know and appreciate my figure again and these new features would take a bit of getting used to.

I was fortunate that I didn't get morning sickness, just mild nausea. It was that kind of travel sick feeling, which I personally think is a different sensation to the sickness you feel if you have a tummy bug. I can cope with seasickness. I've had to run around boats tying knots and moving equipment enough times to be able to function whilst feeling slightly sick. Nonetheless, it's wearing, not simply for a few hours on a boat trip, but for weeks on end.

On top of that, I also suffered from intense exhaustion for the first four months. When I got home from work at around six o'clock I would simply fall unconscious and have to be woken up for dinner. I struggled to work in the evenings, which was often essential as a school teacher. I just didn't have the energy for anything, where before I had always been intensely active: working full-time, playing in a band and karate training three times a week.

No amount of sleep was ever enough, I was constantly exhausted. I had to rewatch TV programmes as I would fall asleep and miss great chunks of them. Unfortunately, because I wasn't continually being sick, everybody thought I was having a great pregnancy, but I felt dreadful and wanted to stay in bed all the time. It's incredibly annoying to be told you are *so* lucky and should be *so* grateful when you feel awful inside. I think pregnancy is tough for everyone. It isn't a competition (although I sort of wanted it to be, one where I would win the title for being the most tired person in the history of the world).

The days passed by quickly and it was soon time for a major milestone, the first scan, at about twelve weeks. I had anticipated this day in excitement because I would get to see my baby. A small part of me still wondered if it was all my imagination and, perhaps, we would find there was nothing there. At no point so far had any medical professional confirmed my pregnancy. They had believed my single positive pregnancy test. What if the test was faulty? I fully expected the sonographer to tell me the whole thing had been some cruel joke.

The day arrived. Despite the nerves in my tummy I had to go into work in the morning. One of the benefits of being a teacher is that you are so busy it's a distraction from things in your life outside of school. I could periodically forget today was 'scan day'. But then it would flood back and my insides would lurch with nerves.

For the early scans it's imperative to drink vast quantities of water so your bladder will push your womb up, out of your pelvis, and make the images easier to see. I was advised to drink around a pint of water an hour before the scan. To be on the safe side, I drank a pint and a half at work and then tried to force more down on the drive to the small local hospital. Stuart met me in the car park. Excited and nervous, we walked towards the ultrasound room with me trying to ignore the enormous pressure from my bladder.

The appointment ran late and so I was not only bursting from excitement but also because I needed a wee. This took the edge off the nerves as my biological urges were more pressing. When we were called in I lay on the bed and pulled up my top. The lady asked if I would pull down my trousers and knickers really low (to my pubic line), I assume because my womb hadn't risen out of my pelvis yet. After smearing some clear, cold gel on to my belly she placed the ultrasound device on me. She pressed right on my bladder, but suddenly there was only one thing in my world.

There, on the screen, was my baby. I was stunned. I at least expected it to take a little searching of grainy images I didn't understand. I spent the next ten minutes getting a tour of my baby's tiny, seventy-two millimetre body, even seeing the miniature walnut brain developing inside the skull. I was surprised to see the baby get thrown around inside of me every time I laughed or spoke. I felt sorry for the little mite as this must be how it spent most of its days, on a continual roller coaster ride.

After a few quick blood tests we left the hospital clutching the first pictures of our baby. I had three beautiful shots, one of which I couldn't make out and had to get Stuart to point out the different body parts. Finally, my baby was real. Not only that, but the risky first trimester was officially over and I could tell the world! Within hours my scan pictures were on Facebook and I excitedly awaited the stunned comments and 'likes'.

It was thrilling when the first signs of a bump appeared. I'd been eagerly anticipating this, as, like many girls, I'd often shoved a cushion up my shirt to see what it would look like. My bump took its time to appear, finally showing itself at around sixteen weeks. To document its expansion I took pictures every week.

I hadn't told my students that I was pregnant because it seemed a bit too personal that early on and because it could serve as a distraction (with attempts to divert the course of a lesson by engaging me in baby talk). But, once my bump showed, the braver, more loquacious of my charges started asking me if I was pregnant. The gossip grapevine resulted in all the students knowing immediately.

The second scan (at around twenty weeks) came along and the big question of gender reared its head. I didn't want to know. I would rather have that 'it's a…' moment. However, Stuart said he would like to know for practical reasons. It hadn't occurred to me he would want to find out the sex of our baby beforehand. I felt he had as much right as I to an opinion on the matter and, as I thought more about it, I realised my curiosity was roused too. If the sonographer knew, I wanted to know.

I had been sure from the start I was having a girl. Other people said different things based on various old wives' tales. What concerned me was that if I didn't find out and got more fixated on the idea of a daughter, I would perhaps be disappointed with a son. Not that I didn't want a boy. Much as it is gender stereotyping, I'd started to dream of dresses, pigtails and dollies and I didn't want that to lead to any false expectations. I wanted to be thrilled either way.

Anyway, there I was on the same chair, covered in gel, when the sonographer asked, 'Would you like to know the sex?'

'Yes,' I breathlessly replied.

8

THE WORLD WE FEED IN

The society we currently live in, shaped by history and culture over thousands of years, is far from perfect, including when it comes to breastfeeding. Events of the last century or so have resulted in breastfeeding becoming a minority practice, usurped by formula milk.

The first commercial infant formula was 'Liebig's soluble food for babies', introduced in 1867. This was a mixture of flour (wheat and malt), cow's milk and potassium bicarbonate.[1] It was initially a liquid and then a powdered form was developed.[1] It became so popular that it wasn't long before other companies followed suit and twenty-seven different types of patented infant foods existed by the end of the 1800s.[1]

In America, in the late nineteenth century, doctors started to recommend the 'percentage method' of concocting infant feeds. Each baby would be given an individualised recipe of milk, water and sugar.[2(p98)] Sadly, the laboratories that produced the mixtures commercially were inaccurate and unclean.[3(p217)] Mothers who tried preparing the complex recipes at home had to return to the doctor to have their formulas modified every few weeks.[3(p217)] It's no wonder this personalised service fell out of fashion.

Evaporated milk was widely available in the early twentieth century.[4] Its use was supported by paediatricians and it became a commonly used infant food.[4] It could be stored safely in a tin at room temperature, which was obviously convenient. Sweetened condensed milk later became popular, even though almost half of its content is sugar.[3(p229)] It was only in 1977 that it was no longer labelled as being a suitable infant food.[3(p230)] Neither of these products was ever nutritionally suitable for babies.

By the 1940s commercial formula was seen as safe and scientific, even considered to be superior to breast milk; an elite substance.[5] Doctors advised using formula, which only improved its reputation.[5] As a result, formula companies increased their advertising to health professionals, and ultimately, to mothers directly.[5(p57)] By the 1970s only a quarter of babies were breastfed by the time they were a week old.[5] In a short space of time, breastfeeding had become a rarity and we found ourselves in a bottle-feeding culture.

Modern formula milk is designed to be similar to breast milk, although it's usually derived from cow's milk, modified to mimic human milk.[6(pp203-204)] It generally contains proteins (whey and casein), fats, vitamins, minerals and lactose.[6(pp208-209)] This is variable depending on the manufacturer and there are special formulas to cater for allergies. For example, soy-based formulas exist for babies who are allergic to cow's milk. There are even 'hungry baby' formulas which are harder for babies to digest and keep them satiated for longer.

Formula can be bought as a powder or as a pre-prepared liquid. According to NHS advice, powders need to be added to recently boiled water (no more than thirty minutes of cooling) since they are not sterile; water of at least 70°C is needed to kill all bacteria.[7] This mixture can then be cooled to a suitable temperature for the baby to drink from a bottle. It's important that the powder is measured, so the amount of nutrients is accurate, and, therefore, formula tins contain a measuring scoop.

Researchers continue to try to make formula milk as similar to breast milk as they can, but it's impossible to copy the way breast milk continually changes, or the live components like antibodies and enzymes. There are so many different specific antibodies and enzymes in breast milk, that change all of the time depending on need, it would be impossible to replicate.

Formula-fed babies feed differently. Since breast milk changes throughout the day, babies will feed in different patterns.[5(pp83-85)] Formula is always the same and so formula-fed babies tend to be more predictable. Formula-fed babies usually also feed less often because it isn't as easy for a baby to digest formula milk.[5(pp83-85)] They might even feed more quickly.[5(pp83-85)]

So, if a mother talks to her friends (who might mostly be formula feeding) then she's not comparing like for like. She will hear about babies who feed regularly, quickly and with long gaps between feeds. If she's comparing that with a breastfed baby who frequently asks for food, it will seem like her baby is starving hungry all the time and demanding instead of biologically normal. It can be extremely damaging for a woman to think that her baby is different, that 'something is wrong' or that formula makes for a more settled and predictable baby. Formula-fed babies seem like the norm and so our biological method of feeding becomes fraught. When you're tired and unsure of yourself it's easy to be swayed.

This is made worse by advertising from companies making the formula milk. In the past (and still in some countries) hospitals gave away free formula samples.[3(pp263-266)] Formula company employees gave gifts to nurses and doctors to encourage them to endorse their products.[3(p238)] Nestlé even notoriously dressed up its saleswomen as nurses in Africa to get poor women to use their products, thinking they were recommended by health professionals![5(p267)] Even now, formula companies spend something like 10-15% of their profits on advertising and many unethical practices continue.[5(p267)] As a result breastfeeding rates have plummeted.

In the 1970s reports appeared that babies were dying in the developing world due to the use of formula.[8] If you don't have access to boiling water then you cannot sterilise a bottle or ensure bacteria present in the powder are killed. Poor women would even often dilute formula to make it last longer, meaning its nutritional content was lowered.[3(p118)] If you also consider that some women may have been illiterate, and so unable to read the instructions,[3(p118)] or even that they may not have been present in her native language[3(pp269-270)] you can see just how hard it would have been to make formula safely for all babies. In these instances the choice between breastfeeding and formula feeding becomes life or death and so the undermining of breastfeeding to sell a product becomes…somewhat unethical.

People started to hear about the aggressive marketing ploys (particularly by Nestlé) that compromised breastfeeding and promoted formula use and they weren't happy. The Nestlé boycott started in 1977[3(p246)] and is still going now in the UK.[9]

In 1981, an ethical marketing code was created to regulate the formula companies and this continues, with the selling of formula milk being restricted by the International code of Marketing of Breast-milk Substitutes. The code states, for example, that infant formula shouldn't be advertised, promotional samples shouldn't be given to mothers or health workers, infant formula should be clearly labelled (preferably including information on breastfeeding), and packaging shouldn't idealise the milk.[10]

While the UK has accepted a lot of the recommendations, the US still hasn't. In fact, only thirty-nine countries have comprehensively implemented the recommendations of the code.[11] In the US, formula is still advertised and women still get given free formula samples in hospital. The Women, Infants and Children (WIC) Food and Nutrition Service still give out free infant formula to low-income families. It gives out so much that they purchase over half of all formula in the US.[2(p207)] This may seem like a nice thing to do, but if you're given free formula you are more likely to turn to it in tricky times rather than seek breastfeeding support.

In the UK, it's illegal to market or promote infant formula in any way.[12] There can't be any adverts, it can't be put on sale, you can't receive loyalty points for its purchase and promotional events aren't allowed. Still, it doesn't take much to find marketing that goes against the code in the UK, even though we supposedly follow it. Also, the formula companies' use of follow-on milks to flout these rules makes me angry. A follow-on milk is one that's aimed at babies over six months old. Since follow-on milks are not for infants they're not technically subject to the same regulations. There is, however, no need for these milks other than to get around marketing rules.[13] Infant formula is sufficient for formula-fed older babies.

One particular TV advert shows the early days of breastfeeding in a muted palette and then, once the follow-on milk is introduced, everything is suddenly depicted in bright, sunny colours. Another shows formula feeding and breastfeeding mothers being at war with one another and, funnily enough, the ones aiming the insults are the breastfeeding mothers. Many show laughing, chubby babies and happy, attractive parents whilst making claims about how this milk is so good for the baby. Due to the nature of my internet browsing I get pop-up adverts all the time for follow-on milks from various brands. Imagine if the reason these adverts were popping up was because I was searching for help with breastfeeding problems! I also object to statements that start along the lines of 'once you are ready to move on from breastfeeding...' You don't need to 'move on' from breastfeeding in this way. Using infant formula is not a given in a baby's life. You can go straight from breast milk to no milk; formula is not an essential stepping stone on the way.

Unfortunately, it's in the formula companies' interest to undermine breastfeeding. Suffice to say, when you are surrounded by formula feeding mothers, your peers tell you how much easier formula will make things, and you see adverts for how great formula milk is...it causes problems. It's more insidious than I realised. I have become very choosy about what companies I am willing to give my money to.

Advice from health professionals is a problem too. My own mother talks about being told in the 1970s to wash her breasts before feeding each time and to set a timer so she didn't feed for 'too long'. You can imagine how undermining this advice can be; I would soon have got fed up with it. Thankfully, expert opinion has moved on. But the fact is that lots of doctors still can't give good enough advice and support. They hardly get any training on breastfeeding and too many think formula and breast milk are equal.[2(p114)] Quite simply, doctors aren't necessarily the right people to turn to when issues arise. Some hospitals have lactation consultants to fill this gap, but not all of them do.

To try and get back to a time when women supported and passed information to each other, a group of women in the US set up La Leche (pronounced 'le-chay' as it's Spanish for 'milk') League in 1956.[14] Women attend meetings where they offer one another support and information about breastfeeding, from mother to mother. Since then, other charities such as the Association of Breastfeeding Mothers (ABM)[15] and the Breastfeeding Network (BFN)[16] have also set up peer support programmes. To my mind, these organisations are leading a cultural change back to when information about breastfeeding was passed through family and friend networks, not through doctors and the media.

Western societies hide breastfeeding; women aren't often seen breastfeeding in public and when they are it's often very covert[17] Breastfeeding in public is legally protected in many parts of the world.[5(p241)] In the UK, it's protected by the Equality Act (2010) which treats it as discrimination if a woman is not permitted to breastfeed.[18] In America it's legally protected in all states, with Idaho being the last state to pass legislation exempting breastfeeding from indecency laws (in 2018).[19]

But even if you are *legally* allowed to breastfeed in public, it doesn't necessarily mean you feel comfortable to do so. Breasts have come, in recent Western society, to be viewed as primarily sexual; other cultures may prefer other body parts such as hips or legs.[3(p146)] We're exposed to busty fashion dolls when we're children, lingerie adverts are commonplace even on roadside billboards, and dressing in low-cut clothes is viewed as sexually provocative. Men will make comments about women's breasts ('Look at the rack on that...') and I've heard men talking in a way that demonstrates that they view their partner's breasts as their sexual property. Some women cosmetically change their breasts to make them appear more sexually appealing, often meaning they can't breastfeed any babies they have in the future. We are told, over and over, breasts are to do with sex and attractiveness.

So, if breasts are part of a sexual identity, and part of sex itself, then it's no surprise that many find it uncomfortable when they are being openly used to feed a baby. This is hard for a new mum to deal with. She may know her rights to breastfeed in public, but if society is unsupportive then that's quite another thing. Not every mum will brazen it out past the looks and comments. Unfortunately, some mums see this as a barrier to feeding altogether; they never try. Others find breastfeeding increasingly difficult as it restricts their freedom to leave the house and so they turn to formula.

When we don't often see breastfeeding we don't get a model for it.[17] When we combine this lack of exposure to breastfeeding with the poor advice we are subject to, it's no great surprise that women struggle with the techniques required to feed their babies. Let's face it, when girls play with dolls we rarely see them hold the doll to their chest to feed it, but almost every doll comes with a bottle to play with. These girls are just mirroring what they are exposed to. In traditional societies, women see breastfeeding regularly throughout their lives and so they learn useful tips from one another.[3(p35)] The more you see breastfeeding, the more normal it seems. It takes the novelty value out of it. It starts conversations that we learn from.

Where do we get information from then, if not from each other or from health care professionals? If we're not talking about breastfeeding with our peers or seeing it taking place then we need to learn somehow. We get a lot of information from TV and the internet. Unfortunately, in the media, formula feeding is shown as an everyday occurrence, while breastfeeding is seen as a novelty.

Think about the times when you've seen breastfeeding discussed on a chat show (often with a polarised phone-in) and compare that to the number of times you've heard formula feeding being treated in that way. When you're watching programmes look out for the number of babies being fed with a bottle compared to those being breastfed. It is quite shocking once you start noticing. Breastfeeding is often portrayed only to discuss the issues with it. I've seen whole programmes dedicated to the shock value of women choosing to feed for extended periods of time, which surely only serves to polarise and, unfortunately, possibly disgust. Even comedy shows poke fun at how 'embarrassing' breastfeeding is. For example, the word 'bitty' from the British TV comedy programme *Little Britain* (a word used in the show by a grown male character to his mother when he wants breast milk) is all too often used as a 'joke' or an insult towards breastfeeding mothers.

Books on breastfeeding can be inaccurate or out of date[3(pp43-44)] (especially if, like me, you raided your mother-in-law's old pregnancy books that were full of advice that has since been proved wrong). New research is always being published which changes our understanding of breastfeeding. It takes time for that to reach advice books and for old books to be discarded.

The internet, of course, is a minefield as with any subject. Information can be wrong, biased, out of date…or perfectly accurate. You need to know where to look and who to trust. The Facebook decency code, all too often, results in pictures of breastfeeding women being taken down (even on private support groups) whilst sexual, offensive and disturbing images seem to appear on far too regular a basis.

I could go on. The media as a whole portrays breastfeeding as out of the ordinary. If you don't think that it's normal to breastfeed, if you think that most people don't do it, or that people who do it have issues or are weird, then it adds to the assumption you that might not be able to, or want to, breastfeed.

I'm sure we've all heard the 'breast is best' slogan (although it's fallen out of fashion amongst breastfeeding mums). In general, people seem to think breast milk is 'better for you' and formula milk is 'unnatural'.[20] There is also a public attitude that breastfeeding is linked to being a 'good' mother.[21] But this all leads to a situation where mothers who have 'failed' to breastfeed feel inadequate.[22] The word 'fail' alone labels women in a horrible way

It's not only if you stop breastfeeding, but also if you struggle, then you start to question your mothering ability because breastfeeding is so wrapped up in our social perception of being a good parent. Since we're told breastfeeding is the best possible thing we can do for our baby, if we can't manage then that has a serious impact on our maternal confidence. It also breeds the kind of tension that sometimes exists between mothers who breastfeed and those that don't.

But when we're up against years of breastfeeding being undermined it shouldn't come down to feeling like you're not 'good enough'. When we are constantly told how wonderful breastfeeding is, while society is distinctly lacking, it feels like we're setting women up to fail. Until rates of breastfeeding rise sufficiently for women to, once again, start to spread their knowledge and experience extensively through their networks, we can't expect them to breastfeed simply because we tell them it's great, and then make them feel bad if they don't.

Equally, if breastfeeding doesn't stand up to being the wondrous thing we've been told it is then we're likely to feel undersold and demoralised. Surely, it's a far healthier situation if we're informed of the realities of breastfeeding and supported through the challenges of the societal pressures we face? Something has to change. It is wrong that breastfeeding should be made so hard. But it's also wrong that *not* breastfeeding is loaded with blame.

Breastfeeding is a fundamental part of female mammalian biology and if we really care about rights for women then this is a pretty good place to begin.

9

PREPARATIONS

I looked at the image dancing on the screen to see if I could tell whether the baby was a boy or a girl. The sonographer tried to see, but the scar from my belly button was lying across the baby's middle forming a dark shadow, whatever angle she tried to look. After taking lots of measurements she said, 'OK, let's have another look and see if baby has moved.'

Stuart and I waited breathlessly, taking little nervous glances at each other. 'Let me see...Yes, that looks like a boy to me.' Stuart (who had said 'boy' all along) looked at me with joy in his eyes. I was shocked. I'd been so certain I was having a girl! Perhaps it would be a good idea to start thinking of some boys' names.

My bump didn't get big quickly. It was solid and completely 'full of baby' (not much water or fat) so I was surprised it was a while before I felt the first fluttery movements. I thought, without much room in there, there wouldn't be much space between fidgety little feet and my nerve endings. But, slowly, I began to realise that what I'd thought was gurgling from my digestive system was actually wriggling. I was desperate for Stuart to feel the movements too and once they were quite strong he was able to. It's a magical moment to share. Eventually, I spent most days being beaten black and blue by the little guy. He liked to wedge himself with his head right up in my ribs and his legs firmly against my hips so that every movement would be particularly annoying. He got hiccoughs daily and would ricochet off various organs with each spasm.

I began to feel my bras were tight so I went to get measured. I expected maybe to have gone up one size. I had, however, already gone from a C to a DD! By the end of my pregnancy my breasts were enormous. Although they were in proportion with my bump I was rather shocked to become an F cup.

I wasn't keen on how much bigger than usual my breasts were. It also seemed hard to get nursing bras that had any padding or support on the high street. I purchased a couple of thin, fabric nursing bras feeling miserable at the prospect of never having my normal chest again (although, of course, I would in the fullness of time).

The first antenatal class I attended was a day about breast-feeding. When I asked work for the day off my boss was surprised that breastfeeding could take up a whole day. To be honest, I was fairly surprised myself, but I was up for anything that bought me a day off work in term time.

We had been instructed to bring dolls with us to practice, so we all turned up with our oversized handbags hiding dollies and teddy bears. Mine was the baby doll I had played with as a girl, which seemed symbolic in some way (even if it was terrifying with eyes that opened when you sat it up). I felt reasonably convinced it was the size of a new baby. I'd previously secretly held it and laid it in the Moses basket to help imagine what things would be like with a real baby.

All of us mums-to-be were nervous and uncomfortable in our later stages of pregnancy, although I wasn't quite as far along as some. The midwife, Ruth, running the class had a kind face and a beautiful, melodious and gentle voice. She reminded me somewhat of the lovely Moira Stuart. I could have listened to her for days. Ruth must have been absolutely amazing during labour. Her dulcet tones complemented the compelling stories of breastfeeding she began to weave.

I had always intended to breastfeed without even really thinking about it. I don't know why. My mum had breastfed me, not that I remember particularly talking about it with her. I tend to lean towards natural methods with everything else in my life so breastfeeding, I suppose, was a 'good fit'. However, any baby I'd ever had any contact with had been bottle fed; I had bottle fed my sister and a little girl my mum used to child-mind. Nonetheless, I had assumed I would breastfeed. Despite my intentions, it transpired I knew little about it.

Ruth explained the benefits of breastfeeding and skin-to-skin contact as soon as possible after birth. Laying a baby's bare skin on your own can help to initiate breastfeeding by stimulating hormones.[1(p22)] In fact, if you give it a chance, the baby will instinctively crawl its way slowly up to your breasts, find the nipple and begin to feed (the 'breast crawl').[1(p56)] I suppose, in this scenario, the baby teaches you how it's done. It puts me in mind of baby turtles crawling to the sea. When I worked on the turtle conservation project we were instructed that baby turtles had to be placed on the beach and allowed to crawl down, rather than put straight into the sea.

Ruth also told us all about how our milk works and it opened my eyes to the fact that this mammalian substance, which I was used to seeing homogenous in bottles having come from another species, was actually a living, changeable liquid. My body could make this fluid that was the perfect nutrition for my child. It was fascinating. I wanted to know more.

As the day continued, Ruth described feeding on demand and explained why the old scenario of feeding at regular intervals existed. A friend had recently had her second baby and I'd seen her frequently feed her children. I had confidently told Stuart that I would make my child wait and get into a routine. I felt she was pandering to her babies and making things difficult by not making them wait. But it seems I'd been a victim of the cultural pressures I've already discussed. Following the cues of a breastfed baby maintains milk supply and meets the needs of the baby's appetite.

It seems my friend had been absolutely right, whereas I had misconceptions that had leached into me from a society that doesn't understand how breastfeeding works. This was my first introduction to the politics of breastfeeding. Up to this point, I had no idea there were politics surrounding the subject. I thought you simply chose to breastfeed and got on with it.

This was the moment I started to notice that not everything was hunky dory in the world of infant feeding. I was shocked that, at one time, mothers were forced to wait with screaming babies for the correct time to tick around before they were supposed to feed them, like my own mother. Despite our understanding of how breastfeeding works having moved on, these ideas still linger in society.

The final section began with a basket of knitted breasts being passed around and each of us choosing a breast. There were big ones and small ones, pale flesh tones and dark. Most mums seemed to be trying to get one similar to their own and so lots of giggling and kindly teasing ensued. With these cuddly breasts we were taught how to massage to stimulate milk flow. So there we were, twenty or so women in the late stages of pregnancy, massaging knitted boobs. I felt embarrassed and flustered and I can only imagine that the others were too, it was so ridiculous (although, I hasten to add, useful). I looked around and realised everyone else was holding their boobs against their chests, mine was lying in my lap (and as yet they haven't sagged quite that far). I went scarlet as I realised my mistake, and quickly held mine up to my chest hoping nobody had noticed.

We then had to hold our dolls up to our bodies in a cradle breastfeeding hold. I was surprised it was in any way different than when a baby is bottle fed. I had to be corrected (surprise, surprise) as I am terminally uncoordinated. Having said that, once I'd been shown, it was straightforward and I felt confident in lining my baby up so his nose was level with my nipple and his belly laid flat across my own.

I left full of fascination for lactation and with an absolute certainty I would be able to breastfeed as I'd now been told everything I could possibly need to know (as if). I came home raving at Stuart about how interesting it was.

A seed of thought germinated over the coming weeks. Why did we need to go to a class? Women the world over manage to breastfeed their babies without having special lessons with dolls and knitted boobs. Why did I struggle and feel so unfamiliar with techniques that were normal to millions of other women?

I was familiar with bottle-feeding real babies. I'd also fed a multitude of dolls in my younger days with a bottle. Not once had I ever played at breastfeeding, I had seen many, many women bottle-feeding babies but I had only seen one friend breastfeed. I was twenty-six years old and rarely seen this most ordinary of mammalian behaviours in my own species! Women around the world see members of their families and friends breastfeeding their babies; they pick up little tricks of the trade. Later, when it's their turn, that helps them to have some idea of what they need to do. It seems I had missed this. There should be no need for classes (although I'm glad I had the opportunity or I would have floundered without a clue). You can rest assured I shall explain a thing or two to my daughters and actively point out any woman who is breastfeeding.

As a biology teacher, how on earth had I never taught this at school? I could see the value in teaching something like menstruation, for example, to ensure teenagers have some understanding of why half the population bleeds once a month. But then, menstruation will happen without any input from you. Lactation, on the other hand, another biological phenomenon that affects around half the population, requires some understanding of how it works in order to do it. It's a learnt behaviour.[2] That is left off the curriculum? Surely, preparation for parenthood is vital at school? Since lactation is fairly central to our biology should it not be a priority to learn a little about it?

I also began to wonder why that class was women only. There wasn't anything that was exceptionally embarrassing, especially when compared to the antenatal classes you go to as a couple, which discuss vaginas and cervixes. Surely, it's of equal importance that men can support women breast-feeding. Would it not be of great value for men to be able to understand the biological process going on so they can be supportive partners? It may also go some way towards de-sexualising breasts.

My head was swimming with all these new ideas that needed expansion and consideration. This was bigger than just me feeding a baby. I could feel it was the start of *something*.

One evening I was getting ready for bed and I noticed my nipple was damp. I'd heard about leaking and I wondered if this was beginning to happen to me. I squeezed gently and a tiny droplet formed; a tiny bead of cloudy water. I wore breast pads for a few days to be on the safe side as I imagined a sudden spurt of milk erupting from my now enormous breasts. I was terrified of being in the middle of teaching and having a pupil point out my wet top. I kept checking to see if my pads were wet or if there was any other sign of milk. I was fascinated and couldn't help but keep prodding to see what happened. Although I could still force the tiny droplets out, I never again saw any signs of a leak and so I soon stopped bothering to wear pads. This was good because, it being summer, you could see them through all my tops, which made it look like I had biscuit-sized nipples.

I also had a further day-long antenatal class about the scary bit; the birth. Now, I was ridiculously cocky about the birth. Having competed in a few painful sparring bouts in karate and having had some seriously gruelling training sessions, I was of the opinion that I had a high pain threshold and good endurance. I had nearly been sick in my black-belt grading from fear and exhaustion and I'd survived being kicked in the face, dragged around the floor and generally beaten up over the years (you may gather I wasn't very good at sparring). Surely, birth couldn't be a lot worse? I figured that the women you see giving birth on TV screaming their heads off are wusses and had been chosen to make the programmes more interesting. Many mothers tried to tell me I was deluded, but, as I told them, I would rather live in ignorant bliss until 'B-day' than have nightmares about what was inevitably to come.

I had googled the process of childbirth in huge detail. I had also taught the subject so I was fairly blasé about the whole thing. A bit of blood and screaming didn't scare me. As a result, the antenatal class taught me nothing new and Stuart and I sat in the front row eating our corned beef sandwiches and giggling like silly schoolchildren.

I'd envisioned sitting propped by Stuart with him rubbing my shoulders and breathing with me. I was hoping to learn the breathing techniques you see on television, the kind with the 'hoo-ing' and 'ha-ing'. But, when we asked about this, the midwife leading the day simply said, 'You've been breathing since you were born. You'll be fine.' I can't say I found this particularly helpful, especially since focussed breathing can really help you to cope with contractions. Anyway, I was now apparently educated in the skills needed and ready for whatever was to come.

At the same class, we were also shown around the birth centre which made things remarkably real. I saw the bedrooms with actual cots that newborn babies go in. I saw the real baths that water births happen in. Some of the others had a go at the gas and air but Stuart and I were too shy. Although I didn't want to have my baby at this particular centre, it was the most local. I found it odd that I would soon be living these experiences we were talking about and my own baby would be laying in one of those tiny plastic cots.

There were various options for where to have my baby and I had given this careful thought. We were lucky enough to live near this local birthing centre. It could offer us birthing pools that were rarely available elsewhere, greater attention than in a typical hospital and a more homely environment. They also had double beds so your partner could stay after the birth and you and your baby could stay as long as you needed. However, on the downside, there was only gas and air and pethidine as pain relief, and if anything serious went wrong it was a twenty mile ambulance drive to a hospital with consultants who could deal with the problem.

I visited the hospital too and found they not only had the high risk consultant-led unit (what you would normally think of when you imagine women having babies in hospitals) but they also had a midwife-led unit of their own. The only difference between this and the one near my home being that you couldn't stay for more than twenty-four hours following the birth and your partner couldn't stay.

It seemed to me, on balance, that it made more sense to go to the midwife-led unit in the hospital because if anything went wrong they could wheel me upstairs to the consultant-led unit, rather than having to go in an ambulance, adding time in an emergency. It was also shiny and new with iPod docks in every room. I didn't have an iPod, but I was impressed nonetheless. This was where I chose to have the baby. Our local birth centre was still in charge of my care because this is where our midwives were based, so this was our first port of call should anything occur.

Towards the end of my pregnancy I suffered a lot from Braxton Hicks contractions. They were totally painless, but my bump would go completely solid like a bowling ball. It was weird and uncomfortable, so the regularity of them became an annoyance. I would also start to get nervous in case it was the start of the real thing. I got several bouts each day and, strangely, they would start up every time I drove. Perhaps my driving was so bad it made the baby want to get out? I can't say I blamed him.

I finished work two weeks before my due date, at the end of the school year. I could not *wait* for the beginning of my maternity. The last few weeks had been a struggle. I was uncomfortable standing as the baby dropped quite early and it was painful to walk long distances. This necessity to sit down so much made teaching hard as it's a surprisingly active job. However, sitting on laboratory stools for large proportions of the day and being forced to waddle about periodically made my back ache. Fortunately, my boss gave me a high-backed chair to help. Still, every evening I was sore and tired and I would drive home exhausted with wave after wave of Braxton Hicks. I felt guilty that I wasn't acquitting myself fully at work because I simply didn't have the energy but I was determined to make it to the end. I didn't want to cry off with just a week to go, leaving my students with a cover teacher. The last day came as a huge relief and was highly emotional as all good last days of summer term should be.

More than anything else I'd been looking forward to a good rest, but I'm bad at resting. I busied myself with tasks around the house as well as a bit of nesting. I had everything organised and ready in his room and I had read every book about pregnancy and birth I could lay my hands on. I did those little things I had always planned to get round to eventually, such as scanning all of our old photos into our computer. I thought it was better to keep myself busy rather than sitting about obsessing over each twinge.

Even though there was still time to go I was desperate for the end of the pregnancy as I didn't particularly enjoy being pregnant, so I tried a lot of 'remedies' (although curries and walks were somewhat more appealing than sex at this enormous size). I hoped the baby would come early; I couldn't bear the idea of my pregnancy going on and then having to be induced. I had had enough long before my due date.

One Saturday, I decided to go to Broadstairs Folk Week. By now my mum had moved to Kent and so she came to join us for the day. This festival goes on for a week, with Morris dancers and folk acts swarming and performing on the streets. It was a beautiful summer's day and, in spite of my uncomfortable waddling, we had a lovely time looking around craft stalls and watching the remaining Morris acts as the afternoon's festivities began to draw to a close.

The Broadstairs seafront is on two levels. The bottom level is the sandy beach. Above it there runs a road, beginning at the height of the cliffs with a bandstand and sloping down with a parade of shops and pubs until it meets the beach at the pier. We strolled from one side of the bay to the other down the cliff road. After a feast of fish and chips at the end of the pier, looking out at the beautiful view, we ambled back to the car along the sands, expecting to take the lift at the end of the beach back up to cliff height. We arrived there at ten past six to find, to my horror, the lift had closed at six.

'Right, I'm walking up,' I said.

'Are you sure?' Stuart asked.

'You really shouldn't…' my mum had no time to finish as I'd already started up three flights of steps. Mum was struggling while I strode up (well, I like to think I strode, but it was more of a painful heave) refusing to be beaten. I hoped it might rattle the baby out.

The next morning I awoke at four with a familiar feeling, the ache of my period starting. As the doziness cleared it dawned on me that I was pregnant, so that couldn't be it. My heart started to pound as I realised the poignancy of this sensation. I laid quietly listening to every twinge of my body. An age seemed to pass and then there was that feeling again. It was fairly gentle, but definitely there; a slight tightening of my belly and a slight cramp. Things were about to begin.

10

HAVING BABIES

From the time when I was shoving dolls up my top as a girl to when I was researching my own birth plan as a pregnant woman, I had a developing awareness that birth would happen to me. I think in that respect thinking and talking about it is different for women and men and it can't help but be a feminist issue.

When thinking about birth, before I experienced it, I wondered what my personal experience might be. Sometimes that visualisation might be exciting or romantic. Other times it was frightening, journeying into the unknown. Once you've been through it your thoughts will largely depend on how you feel about your birth experience. It's no great surprise that birth can be very emotive and people have deep-rooted opinions on the best way to go about it.

My image of birth, probably from TV and from talking to women of my mother's generation, was of a woman lying on her back with her legs in stirrups. I can't say I was looking forward to having to do that myself, I can't imagine many would. Fortunately, things are moving away from that scenario with the realisation that moving around can help labour to progress and that lying on your back increases the chances of tearing and slows labour.[1] Being upright allows gravity to help labour progress[2] and is more dignified than having your legs in stirrups.

I may have been over-confident about birth, but there were times when the pragmatic side of me worried about the pain. I'm not alone in that. For centuries there was no escaping it, but the last century or so has brought with it a variety of drugs to tackle this 'problem'. Queen Victoria famously hated childbirth and eagerly used chloroform for the births of her last two babies to mask the pain.[3] In the same way, for many, pain relief is emancipation from something fearful.

For example, in the US in the early twentieth century, women were pushing for access to 'twilight sleep', a form of anaesthesia where women were semi-conscious but couldn't remember what had happened to them.[4] Horrific accounts abound of women being restrained, hallucinating in their beds for long labours that often culminated in assisted delivery.[4] On waking, they would be handed a baby, having no memory of its arrival. Nonetheless, it was women that demanded the right to painless birth.[4] This method is shown in the TV series *Mad Men* (set in the 1960s) when Betty Draper gives birth using 'twilight sleep' while hallucinating and restrained in disturbing scenes.[5] The practice fell out of use in the 1970s following concerns about its safety for babies.[4]

Now, ideas have turned more towards having a 'natural' birth. Women are starting to look, once again, at having babies at home and declining the offer of the drugs now available (which are nowhere near as horrific as twilight sleep).

I suppose now we have medical back up. Where women once died in droves from 'childbed fever' (infections after giving birth) we now know about the need for hygiene and careful postnatal health care.[6] If a labour becomes dangerous, it can be dealt with by doctors. Once upon a time there was no escape from a painful labour. Now, a woman can choose to use pain relief. Historically, hospitals became more popular because they freed women of the fear and very real danger posed by childbirth, even though outcomes were not necessarily better.[7] Now, for some, it can be a safety net instead, allowing women to choose to birth naturally, without fear of the Grim Reaper ever present.

A woman's experience of birth can have a huge effect on her postnatally, including how she feeds her babies.[8(pp123-124)] We could use the analogy of emigrating to another country. Pregnancy would be preparing for that move; choosing somewhere to go, packing your belongings, buying your tickets and so on. Parenthood is your experience once you get there. You can plan a certain amount but you won't know for sure what it will be like until you arrive. Birth is the flight. Time-wise, an insignificant part of the affair, but in terms of experience it's important. Like a flight, some people are relaxed about birth and others are terrified (I've had hypnotherapy for my fear of flying, fortunately, I didn't feel the same way about birth). A relaxed flight sends you excited and happy into your new life. A dangerous or frightening experience might leave you traumatised, struggling to settle in and possibly even wishing you could run back to your old life. Breastfeeding is like the career you've planned when you get there. It's not going to be easy to get up and go to work if you're still having flashbacks to the plane plummeting towards the ground. It's not the best example, but you get the idea.

There are similarities in the narratives surrounding birth and breastfeeding. Like breastfeeding, birth has been subject to social pressures and medicalisation.[9] Both evoke emotive opinions. In both spheres women are looking increasingly back to biological norms. Of course, it's not as simple as saying, 'OK, everyone is having a water birth at home now and we're all going to love it.' It's complex.

In the UK less than half of all mothers give birth vaginally with no interventions (such as forceps).[8(p115)] Over a quarter of babies are born by caesarean section.[10] In the US, this increases to a third.[8(p115)] Now, if this is a matter of women making informed choices about birth that's one thing (and emergencies do unfortunately happen), however, an awful lot of women have avoidable interventions.

Firstly, it's important to understand how birth works. In a nutshell, oxytocin, that love hormone, stimulates contractions (the first stage of labour). It also helps to decrease the feeling of pain.[11] Each contraction stimulates more oxytocin release, so they become increasingly forceful until the baby is born (the second stage of labour). The placenta is then delivered (the third stage), ideally with the help of oxytocin produced by the first breastfeed.

Stress has a detrimental effect on oxytocin release.[12] So, anything that increases stress, such as being in an unfamiliar environment (for example, a hospital), bright lighting, medical observations, stressed out staff and so on can slow labour and result in a higher chance of intervention.[13] The more relaxed and 'in the zone' a mother is, the more able her hormones are to control a straightforward birth.

Some women have assisted deliveries, where the pushes of the mother are supplemented by a doctor using forceps or ventouse (like a hoover that attaches to the baby's head). I doubt that they would appear on a birth plan as a choice for how a baby is born, but sometimes they happen. Of course nobody would object when medical necessity requires intervention, but it's unlikely to leave you feeling empowered and accomplished. It can be a stressful experience for the baby too and can bruise the baby's head making feeding uncomfortable for them.[8(pp117-118)] It doesn't quite lend itself to having the oxytocin flowing to make early breastfeeding easier.

Episiotomy (a small cut of the perineum sometimes used to prevent tearing) is becoming less common as a matter of routine. Cutting a woman as a matter of course seems somehow wrong. For medical necessity, then, naturally, it makes sense. But it has been found that, in some circumstances, it actually makes matters worse.[14]

Caesarean sections, where babies are born surgically 'through the sunroof', as some say, also reduces the rate of breastfeeding.[15] When you're recovering from surgery and suffering abdominal pain it's not easy to keep getting your baby and trying to hold them comfortably. You're likely to want to rest and recover. After a caesarean less oxytocin and prolactin are released so milk production can be delayed.[16] It's also less likely that you get to have skin-to-skin time after birth[17] so that further reduces oxytocin. Babies born by caesarean are also sometimes sleepier which doesn't help either.[18]

Pain relief drugs during labour also have an effect. For instance, pethidine, a sedative, is used by some women. If used towards the end of labour it can make babies more sleepy so it takes them longer to start feeding.[8(pp117-118)]

If a woman has an epidural, a spinal block to numb the pain, she is less likely to successfully breastfeed.[19] An epidural makes it less easy to follow the body's lead during birth, such as moving into the most comfortable position, so birth interventions become more common.[20] It's been found that women who have epidurals have less oxytocin circulating their bodies[21] which may also explain why breastfeeding is less common afterwards.

After birth, women need time and space to recover, bond and start to breastfeed. They need peace and privacy. Ideally, there should be a 'golden hour' where a mother is left alone to snuggle with her baby without being fiddled about with (all being safe medically, of course).[22] The ideal, in terms of breastfeeding is to have the baby and mother together so they can breastfeed at will. In the UK it used to be normal for the baby to be sent to a nursery while the mother rested and brought back periodically for feeds.[8(p130)] This is now a relatively rare practice but, in some parts of the world, including the US, it's still reasonably common.[8(p131)] Some women would prefer this opportunity to recover from birth, however, it has consequences for that early bonding time and breastfeeding.

If a woman is aware of the possible effects of birth options on her decision to breastfeed then she has the power to make the right choices for her. She might plan her labour to give her the best chance to get breastfeeding off to a good start (as much as one can plan these things). These will often also be the things to make birth go as straightforwardly as possible. So she might choose to birth in the place that makes her feel safest and most relaxed. She might try to minimise interventions and pain relief drugs. She might try to ensure that she has as much skin-to-skin time as possible after the birth and that the baby is kept in her room. But also, if things don't go to plan she will understand the possible knock-on effects on breastfeeding. For instance, if she's had a caesarean and her milk is late coming in she won't panic that she has no milk; she will know this is something that can happen.

Often, if a woman has endured a difficult birth, the attitude may be that the baby should be given formula to allow the woman to rest and recover. Of course, it's a hard thing to breastfeed when you want to sleep off an ordeal, but the early days of breastfeeding are very important in establishing that practice. Socially, we need to start to understand that rather than offering to feed the baby for a new mum, we should be offering to take up all the other threads of her life instead. Many cultures have a traditional forty day resting period after a baby is born (including Western traditions where a woman was expected to be housebound until she had been 'churched' or blessed at six weeks post-partum). [6(p37, p40)]

It seems, at least, we are moving away from some of the routine practices of the past. Having to be shaved, have an enema and then put your legs in stirrups is not only going to impede the flow of oxytocin but also not be the best memory of your baby's arrival. Whilst these are, perhaps, extreme examples there are plenty of things that occur during birth that are unnecessarily humiliating. Being given unnecessary vaginal examinations, having procedures such as membrane sweeps without permission... Rather than feeling proud and powerful you're more likely to feel violated.

Instead of being told 'how it's done' we need to understand how our bodies work and then make the best choices we can to optimise our experiences. During birth, rather than being told what 'needs' to be done, we need to be asked permission. A woman doesn't become a walking womb, of no importance but as a vessel of life. In fact, her physical and mental health are an important part of early motherhood. Rather than laying back and accepting whatever she is told to do, she ought to be making empowered and dignified decisions about her own body.

If women are treated as lesser, if they are humiliated and frightened then really, it's not OK. It's not all right to trivialise their experience and say 'well you got a healthy baby at the end of it'. A labouring woman still has the power of consent. She still has the right to be informed of what her choices are and to decide to follow any path she wishes. A woman in labour may be in a primal state, but she is not out of the loop and powerless. In fact she is, at that moment, a source of power and of life.

A good birth can look different for different people. Some prefer hospital and some are more comfortable at home. Some want to feel no pain at all and others find the pain helpful. Some would prefer surgery and some find that frightening. Ultimately a good birth, where a woman feels strong and gets that oxytocin flowing, can lead her to a more successful breastfeeding journey. If a woman can make plans in full knowledge of the consequences of her choices and then be supported to make the best of her experience then that is truly an empowering thing.

11

BIRTH

I got up, grabbed a pad and a pen and waddled downstairs where I put on the TV as a distraction and waited for the next contraction. I wrote down the time of each contraction and worked out the interval between but it was different every time.

I had been struggling to sleep for weeks due to the general discomforts of pregnancy and a dose of restless legs. This was one of the worst symptoms of pregnancy for me. I had a pressing need to move my legs to relieve the weird sensation in them. It's a sort of tingling, akin to when you've done too much exercise. It's quite impossible to sleep or relax and the only relief comes from movement. Of course, if you're moving, you aren't sleeping. My legs would twitch involuntarily if I tried to stay still. I could get some relief by stretching; however, doing 'downward facing dog' becomes progressively more difficult in later pregnancy. It helped a bit to sit in very hot or very cold water.

Stuart would find me in the wee hours stretching or

sitting in baths of freezing cold water. Often I had ended up sleeping on the sofa after falling asleep watching TV to try and ignore the feeling. On this occasion, when he got up for his morning shift at work, Stuart looked at me sympathetically.

'Another bad night?' he asked.

'No, I think it's…it,' I replied, showing him the pad.

'Are you serious? Is it bad?' He looked anxious.

'No, it's all over the place and doesn't hurt much.'

'Should I go to work?' he asked.

'Well, as long as you're available to come home quickly, I guess so.' Stuart would often be unreachable at work and I was used to sending him messages and receiving no reply.

'OK, well, call my work landline if you need to, they can radio me.' Reticently he left for work.

I tried desperately to get some sleep while I waited for him to return. But each little contraction would have me obsessing over timings. I busied myself with finishing photograph scanning and periodically searching the internet for the signs of labour for the gazillionth time. I wondered if it was real because I hadn't had a 'show' (the mucous plug coming out, sort of like pinkish snot) and my contractions weren't anywhere near the five minutes apart mark that I had been told was the sign I needed to call the hospital.

Little had changed by the time Stuart came home, except I was drained. In retrospect, I should have gone to bed. Even if I didn't sleep, closing my eyes would have helped. But I was so sure everything would suddenly escalate that I was too adrenalised to sleep.

Around dinner time the pain was becoming more intense and I struggled to eat, which is serious indeed in my world. I kept pausing for each wave of pain to wash over me. But the contractions were still completely irregular. I'd been in labour all day; surely I must be nearing the end?

To help with the pain, Stuart strapped a TENS machine on to me. This piece of kit sends electric impulses into your back which stimulate the body to produce endorphins, the body's natural painkillers.[1] I felt it was worth a go as some people had said they found this helpful. It felt tingly and seemed to take the edge off the pain. When a contraction hit I had to press a little button which changed the pulses from a regular pattern to constant. I don't know if it was the machine genuinely helping or if it was just a distraction, but either way it did the trick for a while.

As the evening wore on, Stuart decided to get some sleep because he was shattered from his morning shift. Although I'd been unsuccessful in getting sleep there was no real reason for Stuart to suffer too. With uncharacteristic sympathy for his needs I agreed to him getting his head down. Since he thought I would soon be telling stories of how he went to bed when I was in labour, he forced me to sign a release to allow him to do so. I am deadly serious; he wrote it down on a pad and made me sign it.

At about ten I decided I could take no more. I had been on all fours in the living room rocking with the pain. Regular or not, I'd had enough. I shook Stuart awake and we decided to phone the birthing centre. The maternity unit where I had planned to give birth was full so we decided to go the local birthing centre after all. I was a little disappointed, but at least things were moving.

On arrival we were led to a homely, little room. The walls were pale pink and there were light catchers hung from the ceiling. In stark contrast there was a hospital style adjustable bed in the middle of the room and over to one side was the little Perspex cot that looked somewhat like a fish tank with a few blankets laid in it. Here was my baby boy's first bed! In a few hours (I hoped) he would be lying there, brand new. In the corner next to my bed was an old-fashioned, straight-backed armchair for Stuart. We also had a small stereo which we switched on to help while away the hours. One of my regrets is that I didn't bring an mp3 player loaded with music, or a laptop with some films. I'm sure the right kind of music would have helped me to relax.

I was offered gas and air and a birthing ball while we waited for labour to be in a sufficiently advanced stage to be allowed to use the pool. I wanted a water birth and had been anxious about whether a pool would be available. I love the ocean, so it was a natural progression that any child of mine would be born in water.

I declined the gas and air because I wanted to go for as long as possible without any drugs, but I accepted the birthing ball. I was amazed! No longer was I wracked with agony. I was stunned at how it was a comfortable way of sitting, and bouncing helped me to get through the contractions for a good few hours. It apparently also helps to move the baby into a good position for birth.

Finally, I was allowed to go in the pool (this was around six in the morning, over twenty-four hours since I went into labour), and while I waited for it to be filled I started on the gas and air, which quickly masked the pain. The method of taking deep breaths helped me to focus. I took off my TENS machine and put on a bikini ready for the pool.

The water gave instant relief; a lovely, warm supportive bath that helped me relax and supported my big bump. It was like the best bath you've ever got into after a long day at work. It was huge and at blood temperature, a little cool for me since I usually come out of the bath lobster red. However, the rooms were so warm it didn't matter. The room was clinical looking, filled with hospital equipment, but at this point I didn't care much. The gas and air started giving me that giddy feeling you get when you are reasonably drunk.

All in all, things were looking up; I was in a huge bath, basically drunk, and I would soon be meeting my baby. Between contractions I demanded that Stuart feed me fizzy snake sweets to keep up my strength. The contractions were bad but, by rocking on my hands and knees in the pool and taking huge lungfuls of gas and air, I got through them.

The next midwife on shift, Jane, came in to introduce herself. I already knew her from my antenatal appointments. She was talking to me in that slow and patronising way sober people talk to someone who is drunk. I was desperately trying to sound sane but my voice had gone weird and low and I couldn't string together a coherent sentence. I had to talk slowly and concentrate to make any kind of conversation and was prone to giggling fits.

Soon enough I needed to be checked over again and I had to step shakily out of the pool. I felt confident that, before long, my baby would be putting in an appearance. Disappointingly though, things weren't progressing and so my waters were broken. I was barely aware of this occurring; it didn't hurt (that I noticed). Jane had been commending me on how calm I was, but from the moment my waters burst everything changed. Things got hazy and dark in my memory and the pain became all-consuming. I completely lost control of the proceedings. It was like returning to a primal state. I was just an animal.

Back in the water I suddenly felt an overwhelming urge to push. At this point we'd been left alone for a few minutes while the midwives did a shift handover, so Stuart flew into a panic, thinking the baby would show up before they returned. He ran to get them and very quickly they came running into the room with the trolley containing the cot and some other paraphernalia. Jane checked me again.

'I'm sorry. You have a lip of cervix that hasn't dilated. It's still not time to push,' she said. Clearly, my body had other ideas.

'Are you pushing?' she asked. I wasn't sure if she meant that I shouldn't be or reminding me that I should. I slightly lowered my resistance against the urge to push and a wave of muscle contraction took me over. From that point pushing was a complete reflex, like sneezing, and there was nothing whatsoever I could do to stop every muscle in my body tensing to push out this baby.

'You need to stop pushing!' Jane demanded. It was useless. I was desperately trying to relax and gain mind over body but it wasn't working. Resisting contractions was a thousand times more painful than labour had been up to this point. The more I tried to stop, the more I was wracked with tortuous agony. I knew pushing would be a relief, but I wasn't allowed to do it. In the time since, I've done a little reading about this, and I think I should have been allowed to get on with it, my conclusion being that it was unlikely to result in cervical damage,[2] whereas the psychological damage was significant.

I was asked to climb out of the pool one more time, this time I had blood running down my legs. I was alarmed. Jane told me it was nothing to worry about and, although I didn't quite believe her, I tried to remain calm. Standing there dripping water and blood I knew I couldn't cope any more.

I was escorted to lie on the bed again.

'Emma, we need to get a handle on the pain to stop you from trying to push. We can transfer you to hospital where you could get an epidural to take the pain away. What do you think?' Jane asked. I stared at her, unable to speak let alone have an opinion. I'm not sure I could have told you my name. I looked beseechingly at Stuart.

'I think that's best,' he said. I nodded sorrowful consent. I had categorically said I would not have an epidural. The idea of a needle in my spine makes me shudder and I'm aware of the risks, such as an increased chance of caesarean. But all this no longer mattered; I just needed the pain to stop. The enormity of the journey to the main hospital hit me, knowing it was another half an hour of this pain in an ambulance. This was exactly why I'd planned to go the other midwife-led unit and it felt typical that I was now in that predicament I planned to avoid. It was like all my worst birth nightmares were coming true. I didn't want an epidural. I didn't want an ambulance ride. I didn't want a consultant-led unit. I wanted to push in the pool. But I also felt hopeful that soon, very soon, the pain would stop.

The ambulance crew arrived, seemingly within minutes; two fairly young men who were quite blasé about the whole thing. I was horrified that they expected me to clamber from the bed to the gurney that they were going to wheel me out on when I was in such a lot of pain and so huge, but they insisted, so I had no choice (although I protested bitterly).

I was wheeled outside and up a ramp on to the ambulance. Jane jumped in the front, claiming that she gets car sick, and so a paramedic was the only company for Stuart and I in the back.

It was somehow worse being strapped to the gurney because I couldn't move to relieve the pressure. It was about a twenty mile drive to the hospital and my contractions were about three minutes apart. So, if the journey took thirty minutes I might have to tolerate ten more contractions. I wished I didn't know how to count. That was ten contractions more than I could handle. I panicked and said to the paramedic, 'But it's at least a thirty minute drive, I can't do it.'

'No, it's only ten minutes,' he causally replied. This placated me as in my state I completely believed him. Stuart later told me it had been a bare-faced lie. We drove for too long, with the paramedic jokingly telling me not to give birth in the ambulance, and the sound of the siren ever present in the background. Afterwards, Stuart told me that, as I only had on a robe with a blanket over me; my breasts were revealed every time I writhed. He said he kept covering me up, but to no avail as it kept happening. I, on the other hand, had lost all sense of modesty.

On arrival I was wheeled, writhing, groaning and complaining through the hospital, past a sea of blurred face. The relief as I reached the labour ward was palpable. Again I was forced to climb from one bed to another, but I was somewhat more willing as I thought to myself that this was it, someone would stab me with a needle in the next minute or two and everything would be OK. Of course, in my normal state of mind I would know it would take longer than that. I wistfully imagined an anaesthetist with a dart gun.

'The anaesthetist is in surgery right now,' Jane said sheepishly. 'We can give you pethidine to tide you over?' I could have had that without an ambulance trip. I was heartbroken, and torn between not wanting pethidine and being desperate for the pain to go. I was against the idea of pethidine because I knew it could make the baby sleepy and difficult to feed (especially this late in the proceedings).

As I pleaded with Jane for an epidural the hospital midwives prepared a pethidine injection. I felt helpless and as though I'd lost all control of what happened. I knew everyone had our best interests at heart, but I didn't want any of this. The experience was ruined and I hadn't the strength to fight any more.

Jane, having handed over to the hospital midwives, started to make her way out of the room and gave me one last glance as I lay there naked having kicked off the blanket that was covering me. She stopped in her tracks and asked to give me one last check. I nodded. As she examined me she raised her eyes and said, 'You're ready to go.' Never have four words meant so much. Whilst relieved, I was angry I had ended up in this hospital, feeling anxious and frightened, seemingly for nothing. Of course, nobody could have foreseen this happening.

Jane, unfortunately, was at that moment called by the birthing centre and so couldn't stay to deliver the baby. This job fell to the hospital midwives. There were two midwives attending. One, who looked to be nearing retirement, seemed to be in charge and was the only one who spoke to me. The younger midwife buzzed around and had little to do with me.

'Do you mind a student midwife being present?' She asked. I looked over at the young woman with short, blonde hair standing unobtrusively in the corner.

'No,' I managed to say. I had thought a trainee would make me nervous, standing around without much useful to do. But, as it turned out, I didn't care.

The pethidine was forgotten and the mouthpiece for the gas and air was taken from my hand. I started to push, but, ridiculously, after all of that involuntary pushing earlier, now I didn't feel like I could do it. I tried doing what the midwives said, to pull my knees up and drop my chin to my chest and push, but I just couldn't. I heaved over on to all fours and suddenly felt able.

'You'll tear…the wrong way!' warned the midwife. I don't know that this is true…as if I cared. From nowhere I found that last reserve of energy and I determinedly decided this baby was coming out pronto. I would make every push count. I was done with the pain and the frustrations and some control had landed back in my court. That old fighting spirit that had been honed in karate returned. I was angry, scared and frustrated and I knew exactly how to turn that into physical energy. Tiredness and pain were now irrelevant. The time had come.

I used every muscle I had. I was oblivious to what was going on around me. Stuart said afterwards that, at this point, a man had come through the wrong door, walked in and got sworn at by all of us. I don't remember, but I feel sorry for the poor man, goodness knows what the scene was that greeted him. I do, however, remember grim determination and the feeling as each wave of complete tension rode over me. Stuart said you could see every vein in my neck as I pushed with all my might. Afterwards I had a bruise on my chin where some blood vessels had burst.

As the head crowned I decided to try to hold it where it was. There is a certain, two steps forward, one step back, feeling to this part of labour and I was getting annoyed with feeling like every time I stopped pushing my progress was lost. I carefully controlled my muscles. The body control from karate came into force but, before the next contraction hit me, I lost my control and his head retreated again. I was irritated and this made me push all the harder. It was brute force, rage and frustration. The next thing, the head was being born and somebody shouted, 'Vertex delivered!' I heard a little baby whimper and Stuart and I looked at each other in shock. Time stood still as the enormity of the moment hit me.

The voices of the midwife penetrated the fog, 'OK, with the next contraction the body will be born.'

'Stuff that,' I thought, 'I'm not waiting.' I pushed one more time. I don't know whether my contraction was still going or not, but either way the next thing I knew a baby had been passed through my legs and was lying underneath me; purple and covered with blood and vernix (the white waxy stuff).

The time was declared to be 12.13pm, some thirty-two hours since the first twinges of labour. He was crying pitifully as the midwives buzzed around me. There may as well have just been me and my baby in that room, everything else was in soft focus. It's funny the details you recall; I can remember as if it was yesterday the wavy pattern of wet hair on his head. I kept tracing my finger along it while chaos reigned around me.

Much as it's a cliché, there is nothing that can prepare you for that moment. It's completely unique; the feeling of love, hope, relief and exhaustion. All of the pain and anguish is paled in comparison to the bliss of this. It was absolutely the most incredible few seconds of my life. I had been through more emotion and physical demands than ever before and here I was in this perfect moment.

Unfortunately, things weren't over; I still had the third and final stage to go. My original plan was for natural delivery of the placenta. Although I understood that a Syntocinon injection can prevent haemorrhage and also speeds up the whole process,[3] I wanted everything to be natural. I had wanted to breastfeed to stimulate the placenta to be delivered. However, I was advised that due to the length and stress of my labour it would be sensible to get the injection as haemorrhage was more likely. I just agreed. Ridiculously, after hours of agony, I winced and exclaimed as the tiny needle pricked my leg.

The midwife still encouraged me to feed my baby straight away. I had planned to have him placed on my chest, to wriggle his own way to a feed in the 'breast crawl'. However, what actually happened was the midwife grabbed my breast and the baby and brought the two together. I don't remember giving my permission for this, I think all I was asked was if I wanted to breastfeed. It goes to show how exhausted I was that I didn't slap somebody grabbing my breast without my consent. I suppose having been naked and manhandled for hours now it was assumed I didn't mind. But I did.

What a sad state of affairs to have got to a point where I felt no power to choose or protest any more. I think that somebody making you breastfeed without your involvement is a horrid and pointless thing to do. They are my breasts and that was my baby and it ought to be me to connect the two, in order to learn how to do it if nothing else.

It didn't work straight away, but after a few attempts her efforts resulted in him feeding, while I passively watched. It wasn't at all what I had expected. It felt like a hard, painless pinch on my nipple.

This was the beginning of something momentous, but at the time I lay exhausted and shaking, gazing at my son, as the dull ache of contractions delivered my placenta.

12

HOW TO BREASTFEED

It would be great if there could be a fail-safe, step-by-step guide to breastfeeding. There are, of course, fundamental basics, but there wouldn't be the need for the books, resources, groups, classes and discussions about breastfeeding if it was a case of 'follow steps one to five, repeat bi-hourly'. Attempts to reduce breastfeeding to such a formula have been part of the problem. Breastfeeding is an art; it's a dance.

Essentially, a baby is born with a sucking reflex and a rooting reflex (where a baby turns its head towards the stimulus when it's lips or cheeks are touched) which help it to get started.[1(pp56-57)] Pretty much everything else is up to the mother, although even newborn babies can cleverly clamber to the breast using the 'breast crawl'.

The fundamental principles in breastfeeding are positioning and attachment, so, ensuring a baby is positioned suitably to breastfeed and that it's well attached to the breast. There isn't a hard and fast way to do this, everybody is different and breastfeeding is nuanced.

There is no set way to hold a baby to breastfeed, it's really a matter of preference, but a good way to start is 'biological nurturing' or 'laid-back breastfeeding'.[2(pp63-66)] This is where the mum lounges back on a bed or sofa, propped up comfortably with cushions. The baby lies on her body so its weight is on her, tummy-to-tummy. She doesn't have to actively hold the baby, so it lessens arm or back ache and frees her arms. The baby will begin to root for the nipple and the mother can take the lead as much as she feels the need. Often the baby will latch itself on with minimal input. It's a lovely relaxed way to start out.

Another option is to sit, cradling the baby.[2(pp67-68, p72)] Again, the baby's tummy needs to be against its mother's, unlike in bottle-feeding where the baby is more likely to lie on its back. The baby is held in such a way that its head isn't pushed on to the breast. When the baby opens up its mouth the mother can guide him or her into place by pressing gently on the baby's shoulders.

In principle, a baby's nose needs to start opposite the nipple[2(pp63-66)]. Then, when they open their mouth and tip back their head, it puts the nipple at the best angle for the baby's mouth, so the nipple is drawn to the very back of the mouth.[1(pp33-36)]

A baby needs a big mouthful of breast[2(p69)]; I was once told to think of it as the difference between sucking on your finger (which would be the same as nipple sucking) compared to sucking on your arm (which is more like breastfeeding). In the latter you would have more flesh inside your mouth and your cheeks push out instead of suck in.

If the baby is correctly latched on, it should be

comfortable. If it doesn't feel right then the mother can break the suction with her pinky finger and try again. Some women do seem to get a toe-curling pain on initial latch in the early days[1(p38)], but anything that lasts during a feed, or persists beyond a few weeks, needs to be addressed.

One of the things that can make breastfeeding difficult is the inability to know for sure how much milk a baby is getting. Instead, you have to look for signs that milk is being transferred well. The baby will make swallowing noises (which sound like a gentle 'keh').[2(p106)] Its cheeks will be well rounded, the chin will meet the breast and there will be less areola showing below the nipple than above.[1(p50)] The baby should generally seem content. If the baby is feeding noisily, restless, or if feeding is painful then perhaps the positioning and attachment may need adjusting.

The mechanism of latching a baby on isn't the whole story. As I've already said, breastfed babies feed a lot and small babies like to be kept close to their mummies. This means you are potentially sofa bound for a long period. Part of the art is dealing with that. Sometimes your to-do list mounts up and you totally indulge in the baby. Other times you do what you can, perhaps with your baby in a sling or snatching productive moments while they sleep alone. Sometimes other people help out.

Some 'experts' suggest expressing milk at set times and building giving a bottle into your routine, so that other people can feed the baby and bond with it. In my opinion, other people can find different ways to bond with a baby. They can cuddle it, play with it, dress it, change its nappy…you don't need to feed a baby in order to form a bond. Lots of people may want to give the baby a bottle but their time will come, they can give the baby solids, perhaps, or the odd bottle if a mother chooses to express so she can go out. It doesn't have to be regular, unless that's what the mother wants to do.

I understand that some women *want* somebody else to give the baby a bottle and, of course, that's absolutely fine. But there's no *need* to do it. It's not somebody else's prerogative to dictate how you should feed your baby, or to live vicariously through you by feeding your baby. If a woman is breastfeeding then that needs to be respected, not seen as a selfish barrier to other people's relationship with the baby.

Breastfeeding works well as a responsive relationship. By feeding when your baby asks for it you match your milk supply perfectly to their needs, but you also start communicating with your baby. You learn when your baby might need a short 'snack' or a long, relaxed feed. You learn what different feeding patterns mean. For instance, you might recognise that frequent feeding is signalling a baby that needs to check in with you when they are in unfamiliar surroundings, or when they are going down with an illness, or when they are having a growth spurt.

Periodically, a baby will have a growth spurt.[2(p139)] Children seem to grow this way, in sudden bursts rather than as a gradual process. Then you can find yourself sitting feeding a seemingly insatiable baby for hours. If you go with the flow, your milk supply increases to help them grow and then everything settles again.[2(p139)] When you introduce solid food, the rhythm of breastfeeding changes again. It's an intricate dance where the leader can change; as a baby gets older you can communicate with them that they sometimes need to wait.

Given the subtleties of responsive feeding it can be easy to doubt yourself. Without a model of other women feeding around you, it's easy to worry you're feeding too much, too often or not enough. In traditional societies women are more aware of the hurdles to be crossed, or have other women available to reassure them quickly. Western society doesn't work like that so it's important, in my opinion, to establish a support network, a 'village'.

There are lots of breastfeeding support groups, there are phone lines and internet forums. But, equally, if your family and friends are informed and supportive then that's all you need. As long as there are people around to take the pressure off, both in terms of workload and also worries about your parenting journey. Humans are not lone animals, we need communities, however we decide to build them.

Breastfeeding can be hard work. You feed around eight to twelve times every day (and night).[3] We are so used to intellectualising things, but breastfeeding works best when you go with it and don't worry about it. As some say, you wouldn't think about how many times you kiss your baby, so why would you worry how often you breastfeed? It's not just food, it's a physical 'check in'.

There is a lovely blog post I read by the Natural Child Project about why African babies don't cry as much as English babies.[4] The blogger, Claire, noticed that babies are everywhere in Africa but they aren't heard to cry. When

Claire had her own baby, which very definitely cried, she turned to her Kenyan grandmother for advice. Her grandmother told her the answer is 'nyonyo' (the Kenyan word for 'breastfeed'). If the baby complains, no matter the reason, 'nyonyo' is the answer.

Don't worry about the wheres, whens or whys. Nyonyo. Just feed the baby.

13

CRAZY

The feeling of relief after giving birth was, unsurprisingly, huge. The anticipation and fears had been realised and dealt with. The pain had gone. After thirty-two hours, from first niggles to delivery, it was over.

I'd been under the impression that, after birth, I would feel all right. I expected to feel tired and a bit sore down below. Otherwise, I thought I would be back to normal and mooning over my new baby. I didn't anticipate feeling like I'd been hit by a bus, having run a marathon beforehand. My whole body ached and throbbed. But it's true what they say; it was masked by my beautiful baby boy.

'Does baby have a name?' the midwife asked.

'Yes, Finlay,' I answered. It was a name we both liked (and not intentionally due to the shortened, fishy nickname of 'Fin' on my part). One morning, when I was pregnant, I had supposedly sat up in bed and said 'Fin' for no reason at all. We felt it was fate.

As I was examined to see if I needed stitches (I didn't), Finlay was given preliminary checks. Stuart was choking back tears and had the biggest smile. The two main midwives were bustling about doing jobs, but the trainee came and sat next to the bed.

'I thought you were amazing,' she said. I suspect she was a new trainee because she didn't actively do anything during the birth. I wondered if it was her first birth because she seemed touched by the experience. While the others were busy she sat and chatted to me and I was grateful for the attention.

Stuart was instructed by the midwife to dress Finlay. I had offered to show him where to find things in my labour bag and what I wanted our new baby to wear, but he hadn't been interested. I think he regretted that now. He was impatiently searching for tiny garments he'd never seen before, along with the clean clothes and washbag I needed. I took my labour bag and found it all easily.

Stuart began to dress little Finlay. I could see how scared he was of hurting this fragile, squirmy baby. With assistance from one of the midwives, Fin was dressed in a white vest (Stuart was flummoxed by the vest with poppers under the crotch, because it didn't look like the kind of vests he was familiar with), white babygro and white hat. He was then wrapped in a yellow blanket that had been bought by my nana, something special for his first day in the world.

I was offered a bath and gratefully accepted. I was anxious to see my mum and in-laws when they arrived, but it seemed a better prospect if I wasn't covered in sweat and gunk.

The midwife took my washbag and night clothes to the bathroom. I'd agonised about the appropriate nightwear to bring to hospital. All the guides said to bring a nightie that buttoned at the front for easy breastfeeding, but any I found appeared to be designed for ninety-year-old women. I settled for one I already owned that had thin spaghetti straps and was loose enough that it could be pulled down to feed. In case this didn't work out I also had one of Stuart's old button-down shirts.

A midwife showed me to the bathroom, where the bath was already run and my things were arranged. The room was small, dark and unfamiliar and the bath was grimy, due to age rather than dirt I hoped. I felt I ought to be relaxing in the rooftop Jacuzzis of the Bath Spa, not wallowing in this dank hole. Nonetheless, it was the most welcome bath of my entire life. I soaked, rested and restored. The water stung where I had torn during the birth and the water was quickly tinged with my blood, but I didn't care.

I was reticent to linger too long as I knew visitors would soon be arriving. So, as soon as I had washed as best I could and rested enough to brave getting out of the bath unaided, I dressed and dashed (well, painfully shuffled) to see my little boy once more. I was greeted by my in-laws who had already arrived. I was disappointed I hadn't been there to see their faces when they met Finlay. Still, I was thrilled to show off our little bundle to emotional family.

As somebody who is militantly independent, I was surprised that all I wanted after having a baby was my mum. I've never been the kind of person who runs to my mum when I need help, yet seeing her was essential right now. Although my in-laws were sweet, I longed for mum to be there first. The midwives tried to usher me out of the labour room but I refused to go to the maternity ward until Mum had arrived.

Mum's face appeared at the doorway and everything felt better. The hug she gave me washed away some of the previous two days. No words were needed, I knew she was proud, worried and excited all at once. She confessed afterwards that she made a concerted effort to come to me first, rather than straight to the baby, because that's what she would have liked when she had Zack and I. When everybody is so excited about the baby it's easy to feel side-lined, and I am glad my mum made me her priority when she knew I needed to be.

I finally agreed to make my way to the maternity ward. I was sore and unsteady on my feet. I couldn't see straight; everything felt like it was in stop-motion photography, or a flick book. Mum supported me while Stuart pushed Fin in his plastic cot and everyone else followed in a retinue. We were escorted to a clinical looking bed on a shared ward of four, where the three other beds were already occupied. Mine was by the window. I had briefly worked at this hospital after finishing university and I could see the department I had worked in directly below the window and watch the comings and goings of long-forgotten colleagues. I was content enough with my nest and I clambered into bed thankfully. I was given an absorbent pad to put under my bum in case of bleeding and I cocooned myself in the covers.

Soon Laura and her new boyfriend, Richard, arrived. There was the obligatory telling of the birth story and the game of pass the baby. I was in my own happy, spaced-out world. I kept missing snippets of conversation and was really having to concentrate to keep up. After no sleep for two days and all the physical exertion and blood loss, who could be surprised? Pictures taken at the time, show exactly how detached I looked. At the time I thought I was fine, enjoying everyone's delight in Fin.

I began to crave peace so I was relieved when the proposal was made for everyone to go to my in-law's house for a celebratory dinner. My mum and Stuart made noises about staying to support me but I assured them I would be OK and would try to get some sleep.

We were alone, Fin and I. With curtains drawn about our area of the ward we set about getting to know one another.

I tried to relax but it was hard to take in everything that had happened. I kept looking in wonder at Finlay. He was so beautiful, much more so than I had imagined, and he was *real*. I studied his features and tried to remember every little bit of his face and every tiny movement he made. Any time I tried to shut my eyes I was simply too overwhelmed and in love to keep them closed for long.

Soon, Fin started to show signs that he was hungry, exactly like I'd been taught to look out for in the breastfeeding class. He smacked and licked his lips like he could imagine the tastiest dinner. He was doing what he was 'supposed' to do and I had recognised it; I was doing a great job of being a mum. I'd been to the classes and read the books so I would be able to deal with this easily enough. After all, we had both already breastfed once in the labour room. It was going to be easy.

My first experience of breastfeeding had been hurried in

the fugue following labour and hadn't been initiated by me or my baby. Both of us were still clueless as to how to go about it. So this, for me, was the *real* first time.

I ever-so-gently plucked Finlay out of the plastic cot and bared my breast. Even this was a novelty and I was precise about making sure no fabric was in the way. I got comfortable, adjusting the hospital bed so I was sitting up. I laid Fin flat across my arms and lap and then lifted him so he was lying with his tummy against mine, just like I'd been taught to do with my doll. I lined his nose up with my nipple and touched it on his top lip to encourage him to open his mouth. When he did, I quickly brought him on to my breast, exactly as the books, midwives and classes had said. I could scarcely breathe with anticipation…it didn't work.

This didn't deter me one bit, after all, it was our first attempt. I tried again… and again, and again. We were both frustrated and his hunger was clearly growing. The trouble was, *he* hadn't been to any breastfeeding courses. *He* didn't have a clue what to do and actually, in reality, neither did I. Fin had some reflexes and I had some knowledge and a bit of practice with a doll and a knitted breast and, for me, it wasn't enough.

Normally I hate to ask for help. I won't ask where to find the gravy in a supermarket, I won't ask what's in a dish at a restaurant and I certainly won't make any phone enquiries. This even gets to the point where, if I need to deal with something like my mobile phone contract, Stuart makes the call and I simply give my permission. But, since I'd been a big brave girl and pushed something the size of a watermelon out of my hoo-ha with very few drugs, I was feeling very courageous. I decided to be even braver and *ask for some help.* I pressed the buzzer by my bed and listened apprehensively to the sound of approaching footsteps.

A nurse of roughly my own age put her head around the curtain drawn around my bed.

'You buzzed?' she asked

'I think he's hungry. I tried to feed him but…it's not working,' I told her.

'Well, he probably is hungry,' she said, abruptly. I looked at her, not knowing how to respond.

After a pause I said, 'I think I need help.'

'Show me what you're doing then,' she said, and bustled over to look at my bare chest. I showed her nervously my awkward attempts at breastfeeding, feeling uncomfortable at being topless in front of someone I didn't know. Who would have thought I was buck naked in front of a room full of strangers a few hours beforehand?

'Your shoulders are tense. He'll be able to tell, you need to relax,' she admonished. Of course I was tense, this was momentous, difficult and I had a stranger staring at my breasts! She passed me a pillow saying, 'It's for you, not for baby!' Goodness knows what she meant by that. I tried to relax my shoulders and rest my arm on the pillow but it didn't make any difference. The nurse moved my arm a fraction and then disappeared, but Fin still wasn't feeding.

My bravery had achieved nothing. Already I was anxious that he wasn't going to breastfeed. After all my hopes would I fail in the first few hours? I wondered if I would have to resort to formula milk so soon.

It hurt to be spoken to so sharply in my vulnerable state. I had the feeling of standing at the edge of a precipice I never intended to be anywhere near.

I think we're incredibly lucky in the UK that we get a high standard of free medical care from the National Health Service. I came across many wonderful health professionals. I also appreciate that those who are employed by the NHS are overworked, having worked in a hospital once myself. We're all human, not every interaction can be flawless. That said, it was astonishing the effect this incident had on me. I'd expected to receive support in establishing breastfeeding, given how much drive there had seemed to be for it during my pregnancy.

I suppose there were mothers with all sorts of medical issues that mattered more than me. I understand that. I was low risk and low importance. The nurse was probably coming off a long shift or was dealing with much bigger issues than those I presented. I can rationalise all the things that explain that brief interaction and, normally, I would have shrugged it off as rude and moved on with my life. But those few minutes affected me deeply. After so much trauma over the last few days and with the huge weight of new responsibility, I was pushed over the edge.

I felt completely vulnerable, probably for the first time in my life. This little life depended on me and I couldn't even manage to feed him, something totally fundamental and something I had so desperately wanted to do.

I didn't know what I was supposed to do next. I kept trying on my own, but Fin wasn't latching on. I tried everything I could think of, getting increasingly frustrated and sweaty (why are hospitals so hot?) as his cries grew more urgent. I decided to stroke his cheek with my finger, thinking maybe it would help to stimulate his rooting reflex. Suddenly, he moved his head and I felt that pinching feeling again. He had done it, we were breastfeeding! Who needed people? I could manage perfectly well on my own. I was a primitive, independent cavewoman, my cave being made of my firmly drawn curtains around my bed.

Finlay finished feeding quickly. His tiny belly full of my golden colostrum, he pulled away. I changed him to my other breast to see if he wanted more (not that you have to). He wasn't interested.

Having had enough of a conquest for now I put him back in his cot, planning to regroup my emotions. But, looking at Fin, the shock of what I'd been through hit me; all the fear, the pain, compounded by my harsh treatment when I was trying to reach out to somebody. I felt isolated. I realised I couldn't anticipate what was ahead and it seemed like I wasn't going to get a lot of help. Was this the first step on the road of my ineptitude at mothering? I sobbed.

I couldn't stop crying no matter how I tried as I hit this roller coaster low. I texted Stuart to ask him to come back and help me, but got no reply. The anxiety I felt prevented me from calling his parents' home or their mobiles, even though I knew full well Stuart didn't get coverage at their house; I couldn't speak to anybody but Stuart. I felt abandoned and alone.

A breastfeeding peer supporter (a volunteer mum trained to offer breastfeeding support) came to ask if I needed any help and found me weepily starting to pull myself together. I explained I'd struggled to get Fin to latch, without mentioning the nurse. She suggested that when I got home I should try biological nurturing. This made me feel better; it seemed once I was out of this hell-hole I could start again. The peer supporter let the nurses know I was tearful but nobody did anything about it.

The next dilemma wasn't far away; I needed to go to the toilet. What was I meant to do with my baby? I was in no fit state to carry him with me, but what would the nurses think if I left him alone? The logical part of my brain was trying to tell me that mothers the world over left their babies for a moment while they went for a quick wee. But the irrational side of me was panicking that if the nurse saw him alone they would call social services.

I couldn't hold it in indefinitely. There was only one thing for it. I spotted a kind looking nurse dealing with the lady opposite me through a gap in my curtains.

'Excuse me?' I asked tentatively. She looked up. 'What do I do with the baby when I go to the toilet?' I felt my face flush as I wondered if this was actually a stupid question. She looked fleetingly perplexed.

'Leave him there. We'll listen out for him,' she replied. I breathed a sigh of relief.

I slowly got to my feet. As I stood, I saw that both I and my bed were covered in blood. It had seeped into patches not protected by the pad under my bottom and my nightie was soaked. I hadn't anticipated how heavy the bleeding would be after childbirth. In retrospect, I should have checked my mattress-thick maternity pad sooner. I was used to having some notion of how much blood escaped my body but, since my bits weren't feeling like they normally did, I'd lost all sensation of needing to clean myself. I wrapped my dressing gown around me to hide my bloodstained nightclothes, hid the bedsheet under the covers and scuttled off to the bathroom.

On my return I wondered what to do. I didn't have the nerve to ask for new bedding; I'd used up the little courage I had in asking the nurse if I could go to the toilet. The only other thing I had to wear was Stuart's old shirt and it was much too hot for that. Disgusted with myself I decided to live with it. I would be lying down anyway. Nobody need know.

I'd been drinking huge amounts of water, I suppose to replenish my body after the labour. I poured the last drips of water from my jug into my glass and frowned. What would I do? A nurse (a different one again) happened to come and check on me at that moment.

'Could I have some more water?' I asked. With an impatient sigh she took my jug to refill.

Why was everybody so cross with me? I retreated, mentally, further into my bed-cave.

As the evening wore on I continued to experiment with breastfeeding. Sometimes Finlay latched on and sometimes he didn't. I also changed his first nappies. Unfortunately, I hadn't packed enough cotton wool for cleaning his bottom. I was scared to buzz for a nurse in case I got somebody brash again or they thought I was underprepared. Surely, only the most thoughtless mothers didn't pack enough cotton wool. What if they put it on my records and it resulted in me being checked on by social workers? I know it's totally mad to think a social worker would worry that you'd run out of cotton wool, but this demonstrates that I had lost my grip on reality.

No, I was damned if I'd ask for anything ever again. Anyway, I had an idea. Ever enterprising, I went to the toilets and sneakily took a roll of toilet paper. I hid it under my dressing gown and scurried past the nurses' station back to my bed fearing capture. Success!

I took Fin from his cot and started to change him, but it was also getting dark and I didn't know how to turn the light on in my cubicle. I searched everywhere for a switch and came to the conclusion that I must not have a light. Again, I was not in a sensible state of mind, you could see the bulb above my bed. There was a glow from the lights in the corridor and those of the other mums on my ward who clearly did know how to turn on their lights so I managed to get by, trying to time my need for light (for breastfeeding or nappy changing) with those of my adjoining neighbours.

Then came the nuclear poo. Mothers remember that first meconium poo and smile a wistful, amused smile when they talk about it. It was black and sticky, like tar, and it was absolutely everywhere. The beautiful white babygro I wanted Fin to wear for his first day in the world was covered.

Placing Fin on my bed, naively forgetting to use a changing mat, I stripped off his clothes. I piled them at the end of the bed wishing I'd packed a carrier bag to put them in. Removing his nappy, I started cleaning him with my contraband toilet roll dipped in my begrudgingly-given water.

The lady in the bed next to me turned off her light and I was bathed in darkness. Not to be beaten, I rifled through my handbag and found my mobile phone. Switching on the torch, I tried to prop it up so I could see, but it kept falling over. So, with my phone clenched between my teeth I carried on cleaning Fin. Somehow, I was managing to get the sticky, black poo all over my sheets. Since they were already blood-soaked I decided not to worry, I would focus on him.

Just as I finished getting his skin spotless, a fountain of urine soared impossibly high and splashed all over my pillows. Suddenly, my sense of humour returned and I grinned at this ridiculous situation. If anyone had seen me they would have thought I'd completely lost the plot. Smeared in body fluids and cackling with a phone in my mouth, I quite possibly had.

With a new, yellow babygro on, my clean baby went back into his cot. My bed on the other hand was awful. Despite a lift in mood, I still felt I couldn't ask for clean sheets. I turned the pillow so it was urine-side-down and took the sheet I'd been using as a cover and threw it over the lot. I changed into Stuart's shirt, putting my, now, totally disgusting nightie into the pile with Fin's clothes at the end of the bed. I lay on top of my filthy bed without any cover. It was hotter than the sun on the ward anyway.

I know this was disgusting and, in my right mind, I would never behave this way. But, if I admitted the situation to a nurse, I faced the scary prospect of being thought of as inconvenient or worse, inept. I felt I had no other option.

Morning dawned too slowly. Two of the other babies on the ward had cried all night and my opposite neighbour had been buzzing for nurses continually. I struggled to sleep with the constant noise and traffic through the room.

I impatiently counted down the minutes until visiting time began. I wanted to get out of here. I wanted to be home where I was less judged, more clean, had limitless cotton wool and knew how to turn on the lights. It felt like an age since Stuart had left and I couldn't wait for him to come and rescue me.

Stuart called twenty minutes before visiting time commenced and it transpired he hadn't received a single one of my plaintiff texts since he'd decided to sleep at his parents' house. Feeling silly for not realising he might do that, I demanded he come to my aid immediately, but only if he also brought cotton wool and carrier bags.

While I waited for Stuart, a lady from Bounty (a company that offers free samples and markets products to mothers) came round to take pictures of the new babies so you could buy prints online if you wanted. I thought I may as well see how they turned out. I know since then the whole 'Bounty' thing has become controversial since they're marketing products in a medical setting and to vulnerable women[1] but, at the time, I simply thought I'd have some free stuff and nice pictures.

She made a little nest out of blankets for Fin and started to take photos, but the light was all wrong. After several adjustments she said, 'Could you turn on the light over your bed please?' I gazed at her in panic. I would have to reveal my shameful secret.

'I...I don't know how to turn it on,' I confessed.

'Oh? It's that button.' She pointed to my buzzer for the nurse. I was confused. I looked at the console and, just above the big call button, was a small, unmarked rocker switch. Feeling stupid, I pressed the switch and, hey presto, the lights came on.

'Hmm...do you have any more blankets for me to prop him up with?' she asked.

'No, I only brought one with me.' She looked surprised at my ignorance.

'There's usually one under there,' she said, pointing under the cot. I hadn't noticed the little cupboard doors underneath. I opened them to find, not only blankets and a few spare nappies, but also a pile of cotton wool.

It turned out the midwives had told Stuart where everything was (I'm not quite sure why he needed to know) and he'd forgotten to relay the information. Perhaps some labels around the place might have been helpful, but telling a person who isn't staying is of no use whatsoever.

When he arrived I filled Stuart in on the night's occurrences and we had a good laugh since, in the light of day and with somebody to protect me, I was feeling more confident. I proudly showed off my awkward breastfeeding abilities while we waited to be discharged.

I'd been overly optimistic about how much my bump would deflate, so I'd brought a pile of non-maternity clothes with me. Trying to get into the baggy joggers that, pre-pregnancy, were too big, was like getting toothpaste back in the tube. My loose top didn't even begin to pull over my enormous boobs. I had no option but to continue to wear Stuart's old shirt, along with the maternity jeans I'd worn on my way to hospital two days before. Although it was summer Stuart protectively insisted I wear his coat. It reached my knees.

I'm sure I looked crazy as we left, not that it would be a first for me. I did my best not to have a pained 'John Wayne' walk. Still, I was free. Free to go home and try to be the mum I'd hoped I would be.

14

MOST PEOPLE BREASTFEED, RIGHT?

Before I actually breastfed a baby I had no concept of how common, or otherwise, breastfeeding was. I also didn't understand how emotionally charged that decision can be. I thought most people started out breastfeeding and then moved to formula when the baby was bigger. This was before I realised that formula didn't need to be a natural progression. Formula is so commonplace and breastfeeding so rare that it skewed my concept of 'normal'.

The reality is pretty stark. About a third of babies around the world are exclusively breastfed for the first four months of their lives.[1] So, all the other babies get at least some alternative food, mostly formula, in that initial stage. So much for most women starting out breastfeeding.

In fact, in the UK, where I live, breastfeeding rates are among the lowest in the world. The Infant Feeding Survey in 2010 (the year Fin was born) found that 81% of UK mothers initiated breastfeeding.[2] Although this seems a lot, this figure includes babies that breastfed once only or who were given expressed breast milk initially. After a week only 69% were still breastfeeding, by six months just 34% were giving any breast milk at all and a staggering 1% were exclusively breastfeeding, having not given formula or solid food.[2]

In the US, a similar proportion of mothers initiate breastfeeding (71.1%) but at six months 22.3% of babies are exclusively breastfed.[3] Although this is better it's still such a small proportion. It's interesting, given that formula is more freely marketed and in the absence of compulsory, paid maternity leave, that rates are higher than in the UK.[4 (p171)]

Around the world breastfeeding rates are highly variable and reporting is also inconsistent. But, as it stands, only 23 out of 194 countries meet the target of 60% exclusive breastfeeding under six months.[5] It's a global issue.

Lots of people do breastfeed, for a little while anyway, but most of them stop earlier than recommended. There are, of course, hundreds of reasons for why. Some struggle through difficulties with breastfeeding, some lack support or information, some face health issues, some need to return to work… Everyone travels their own path and it's a complex and emotive issue. Formula has a place; we hardly want to be back in the times of babies dying of inadequate nutrition, but breastfeeding should remain the normal way to feed babies.

I'm not saying every woman should breastfeed no matter the consequences; I would champion any woman's right to feed her child however she wants. But, it's heartbreaking that mothers who stop breastfeeding say they would like to have kept going for longer; women who wanted to breastfeed and tried but were unable to continue. When that's because they aren't finding the right support or information it's a sad state of affairs.

There are also many reasons that a woman might not choose to breastfeed at all and she is completely entitled to make that decision. For example, if a woman had suffered some kind of abuse that resulted in her feeling uncomfortable about a breastfeeding relationship, surely only a monster would question that. But whatever the reason, it remains a woman's right to choose how to use her body.

A small percentage of women are biologically unable to breastfeed due to insufficient glandular tissue. Their breasts are characteristically more tube-shaped than the typical rounded breast shape.[4(p66)] Some women may have hormonal issues that wreak havoc with breastfeeding.[6] Some may have had breast surgery, whether cosmetic or otherwise, that makes breastfeeding difficult or impossible. Of course, there are other circumstances that also make breastfeeding challenging such as if a mother is sick, needs to work, or if she dies. Thank goodness we have formula so that these babies can thrive and be fed safely.

There are also other options; in some areas milk banks are available so that women can choose to use human milk over formula, particularly for premature or sick babies in hospital. Women can express and donate milk, having been medically tested beforehand to minimise the risk of infection. Some people set up informal milk-sharing arrangements, which could be questionable given the lack of screening.[7] Although rare, wet nursing still exists, whether it be a formalised, employment situation, or a case of friends or family feeding each other's babies (cross-feeding).[8]

Nonetheless, being breastfed by their own mothers ought to be the more common way that babies are fed, not the minority. Women that started out breastfeeding should, mostly, in theory, be able to carry on doing so. If this were the case then there would be more understanding and acceptance of the practice within society and breastfeeding would become easier for a lot more women. Formula feeding, being arguably a more straightforward process, would be able to continue unencumbered for those that choose that path, but support and information is important for these mums too. One would also hope that people would learn to be less judgemental about the choices women make.

Maybe this is a utopian view, but what I'm trying to say is that too many women have been failed and the problem needs to be addressed.

So few women, so few of my peers, breastfed their babies past early infancy. It's no surprise we find it shocking when a woman breastfeeds a toddler, it's rare enough to feed a small baby.

Despite the fact that, as mammals, breastfeeding ought to be normal, we are just so far removed from it. This is feeding our young, it should be fundamental. A woman struggling to breastfeed due to societal pressures ought to be the headline news, not a woman choosing to breastfeed for an extended (but normal) period of time, or a woman breastfeeding outside of her home.

Ultimately, if part of learning to breastfeed is seeing other women doing it then, at the moment, we're in a self-perpetuating cycle. We don't have the tools learnt through casual observation; we don't feel accepted and comfortable breastfeeding whenever and however we wish. Breastfeeding makes people feel weird; it's a novelty, something shocking or conversation-worthy. But if our generation barely breastfeeds and those that do feel they have to keep it hidden, how on earth are things going to change?

15

BLOOD, SWEAT AND TEARS

Arriving home, we started getting to know Finlay and entertaining hordes of visitors. It was wonderful to see people and show off our exceedingly cute baby but we were so tired.

I spent ages trying to find clothes that looked nice, didn't aggravate any of the tender parts of me, and allowed me to breastfeed. Every time I was left dispirited because I felt fat and unattractive. None of my clothes fitted; maternity clothes swamped me and normal clothes were like *Tubigrip*. Initially, I wore tops that buttoned at the bust. Eventually, I moved on to T-shirts, once I realised I could discreetly lift up my top (and once I'd slimmed down enough to be able to do so).

Perhaps we ought to have put people off for a week or so; our baby was one of the first in our family and friendship groups so people were understandably excited. But having a new baby is overwhelming and entertaining guests isn't always a high priority.

I expected to have piled on the pounds after having a

baby. It seemed reasonable to have gone up a dress size; I'd kept some of my slightly larger clothes for this eventuality. I didn't expect to be struggling to do up clothes two sizes too big. Despite remaining fairly active and eating well during my pregnancy I'd put on far more weight than I realised.

I'd anticipated a deflated-balloon tummy, but I'd hoped the rest of me would be unscathed. You hear mythical stories of mothers who ping back into shape. My mother was one, leaving the hospital in undone, pre-pregnancy, skinny jeans. I thought maybe I would inherit these fantastic genes. Disappointingly, this was not so.

The day after I returned home I decided to have a soak in the bath. I stripped in my bedroom and walked to the bathroom where the water was running. I habitually check my reflection in mirrors I pass, in case I am wearing my top inside-out or have toothpaste on my face (common occurrences). I glanced in the full-length mirror on the landing, something that doesn't even register ordinarily. I stopped in horror. My breasts were enormous, as was my empty tummy. Where was the athletic figure I had once possessed? The disposable paper pants weren't helping the aesthetic either. I didn't even recognise this malformed woman.

Was this it? I'd often heard mothers saying they never got their figure back; would I now forever look like this weird version of myself? After years of learning to love my figure I didn't want to have to readjust my perception of normality to *this*.

I wish I hadn't brought this shock on myself. Your body changes so much in the first couple of weeks following birth that what I saw in the mirror was thoroughly unrepresentative of my future. Even within a week I looked completely different, but I was haunted by that vision in the mirror. Instead of feeling proud of this amazing body that had been home to my baby for nine months and was now still nourishing that baby, I felt disgusted.

I threw myself into weight loss far too quickly. I didn't give myself a chance to recover physically (or mentally). I took my first walk to the shops when Fin was three days old. It was only round the corner but I was breathless from just this little foray. As well as the remaining discomfort from labour, I had clearly lost fitness during pregnancy. Nonetheless, when Fin was a few weeks old, I forced myself to stride around the clifftops near my house. Much as I love walking, this was crazy! I was also soon busying myself with domestic tasks and various projects. I felt a new baby was poor excuse for sitting around when it's probably the best excuse. I wish I'd given myself a break. I should have been lounging about, breastfeeding and recovering, instead of forcing myself to function as if pregnancy and labour had never happened.

Thankfully, my bump visibly reduced every day. I checked it compulsively in the mirror every morning to see the difference from when I'd gone to bed. It helped my ego recover.

As far as I'm concerned, the quick deflation of my bump was due to breastfeeding. Every time I nursed in the first week or two, I got stomach cramps, much like period pains, as hormones stimulated my womb to contract and return to something nearing its original size.[1] I didn't know this happened and so initially I was worried, but a quick internet search reassured me it was normal. Breastfeeding also uses calories.[2] At least if I was inactive because of breastfeeding I could console myself that my body was working to produce food for my baby.

I seemed to sweat away half my mass in the first few nights. I woke up soaked the first night at home. Again, I had no idea this was going to happen but a bit of googling put my mind at ease that it was to do with hormonal changes.[3] It's unfortunate that a lot of these little postpartum things aren't mentioned before you experience them and you can worry unnecessarily

My milk came in when Fin was four days old. I didn't get sore or swollen; I simply noticed my milk had changed colour from a clear fluid to milky-white. Fin seemed more sated too and, after a feed, would fall off the breast and sleep. In these early days Stuart called breast milk 'knock-out juice'. Fin would sometimes sleep for a few hours in a groggy, milky stupor, so I would get a break to read, watch TV, sleep, or, far more commonly, try (unsuccessfully) to do something useful.

I had a gorgeous baby and my body was starting to look less scary. Unfortunately, not everything was rosy in the world of breastfeeding.

Firstly, I had 'latching on pain'.[4] This seems to be something that just happens to some women. I've heard of it being referred to as 'the sixty second sizzle' or 'the toe-curling moment'. All I know was that it hurt. Every time I nursed from day one it felt like I was being stabbed in the breast. I tried to discuss this with my health visitor, but she simply suggested perseverance and had no useful reassurances. I may have given up if I hadn't read some internet forums that said it would only last a week or two and isn't anything to worry about. I couldn't have gone on if I thought that pain would be present at every feed. I decided to dogmatically continue and take a deep breath before every feed.

But, within days of Fin's birth, the pain got worse. As the latching on pain subsided a horrible soreness continued during each feed. My nipples went rough and I assumed this was similar to calluses forming, like when you play guitar, and paid no attention. But soon, my nipples cracked and bled. They scabbed and sometimes, when Fin stopped feeding, I would see traces of blood in his mouth. This was horrifying. I didn't want my baby eating blood.

'If it hurts you're doing it wrong,' I had been told. I didn't interpret this as intended; that pain is a sign you need help. It can be a sign of a bad latch or other issues and it can be fixed. In my strange mind I thought it meant I shouldn't be breastfeeding, that I was doing it wrong. Having problems breastfeeding made me feel utterly useless as a mother. This ought to be instinctive…shouldn't it? I felt like a bad mother, not just a person who needed support (like plenty of other women).

I worried somebody would discover I was breastfeeding 'wrongly' and I would be told to stop. Moreover, the pain was wearing. I had been through labour, a hideous time at the hospital, after-pains, night sweats and now I was bleeding from my poor, sore nipples. How much was I supposed to take? I thought early motherhood was a blissful time, not this panicky, painful, exhausting experience. Was it only me? Nobody told me it would be this hard; I was supposed to be brimming with motherly happiness wasn't I? Everybody was cooing over the baby and telling me how wonderfully we were doing and how lucky I was; why did nobody seem to acknowledge how tough it was?

I was still nervous about asking for help, thanks to my experience in hospital, and I also wasn't ready for the social aspects of visiting the local breastfeeding support group. I worried that on breastfeeding in front of these experienced ladies I would be met with condescension. I thought they would gently tell me, 'This isn't for you, you need to give up.' I worried sick somebody would tell me I had to stop breastfeeding. These experienced breastfeeders would surely spot a fraud like me instantly. I had become so introverted and paranoid it was ridiculous.

Of course, in hindsight, I should have got help. Bleeding nipples are definitely a good sign that you need to seek support. But I'm sure it's evident that I wasn't *right* in myself. My confidence was broken. I shied away from people that could help. I felt I had to hide my problems because I shouldn't be having any. It's not even that I thought people would be unkind; I couldn't bring myself to verbalise my issues, to *say* it was hard. I couldn't admit that being a mum, something I had always wanted to be, was actually really tough.

Fortunately, Finlay wasn't suffering. His weight gain and general health and happiness were fine. If there was some ill effect for him I would have sought help immediately. But for myself? I was willing to just crumble.

It's so important for women to seek out all the support they possibly can from family, friends, health professionals, volunteers…anyone they trust. Had I done this at the first sign of a problem I would have avoided the slippery slope I proceeded to slide down. I could have salvaged the experience of Fin's early days. I wish I had had somebody close who could have recognised those signs that I was struggling to breastfeed and point me in the direction of quality support. Unfortunately, I was on my own.

Instead, I trawled the internet for information. Thank goodness for the internet; heaven knows how women found answers without it. I got Stuart to watch videos of correct latches and then watch me breastfeed and see if it looked right. I was pretty convinced I was doing it correctly since it looked the same as the videos. However, it still hurt.

In the meantime, I was visited regularly by my health visitor. She would ask how breastfeeding was going and I would smile and say it was fine. I avoided feeding in front her and she never asked to see. Once or twice I mentioned nonchalantly that it had been tricky but that I thought I had it sorted now. She wouldn't take the bait. She would tell me I was doing so well feeding him so successfully. Quite frankly I was a good liar. Sure, Fin was happy and healthy, but I wasn't.

Now, I don't mean to suggest breastfeeding mothers should be forced to prove they can do it, forced to feed in front of a health visitor with a clipboard and a magnifying glass, but there needs to be an awareness that sometimes words are just words. I wasn't all right; I was starting to fall apart.

Eventually, my injuries became so bad that one of my nipples essentially split in half. This is exactly as painful as it sounds. I was having to take painkillers to deal with it, which was then making me paranoid about medication leeching through to the baby (in reality, taking paracetamol at the correct dose is no big issue to the baby)[5]. It didn't touch the pain though. I would steel myself to feed on that side, trying to think of anything but the pain when he latched on; perhaps the words to a long-forgotten song, or the alphabet backwards. It was to no avail. I would end up in tears every time, crying out from the pain. Stuart was growing increasingly concerned, which made me try to hide it even more.

'Give Fin formula for a few days!' Stuart said, time and again. Despite my protestations he didn't seem to understand this wasn't an option. I felt breastfeeding wasn't something I could dip in and out of. I knew if I stopped feeding my supply could drop. I had also made my decision that I didn't want to use formula, I wasn't about to change my stubborn mind so soon.

'Ask somebody for help,' Stuart would say. Well, that I couldn't do. Anecdotally, I have heard that often partners (or grandparents) phone breastfeeding helplines for women. This doesn't surprise me at all. Stuart and I didn't know such a thing existed, but I wish we had, I think Stuart would have phoned them in his frustration at my single-mindedness. I know he was at a loss as to what to do about the situation. I suspect he's the only person I would have allowed to seek help for me.

I tried using a lanolin nipple balm to help my nipple to heal but it wasn't doing anything. The worst thing was when Fin latched on badly (which was easy to tell as it would be excruciating), I would have to pull him off and go through the whole process again. I tried icing my nipples before feeding to numb them. Fin was understandably unimpressed. He would mouth at me, pulling faces before he latched on, by which time my nipple would be warm again and so it would hurt anyway.

All in all, breastfeeding was a painful and unhappy experience. I would avoid feeding for as long as I could, frantically delaying the inevitable. Of course, a young baby feeds very frequently. I didn't get to enjoy using breastfeeding as an instant fix. It solves all baby problems: tiredness, hunger, or simply needing some closeness. Instead I had to struggle, rocking, singing, dancing...all while on my knees with exhaustion. I'm sure avoidance was also having an impact on my milk supply and eventually his weight gain, not to mention bonding with Fin and my feelings about my new life. I loved him, but I hated motherhood and breastfeeding.

I was frightened of being forced to give up breastfeeding, although lots of people 'reassured' me that it was OK if I did have to. As soon as I bravely mentioned any difficulty the answer from those around me was to give Fin a bottle, rather than for me to be escorted to a support group or for someone to pick up the phone to a helpline. Of course, it's OK to give a bottle. It's absolutely fine to formula feed if that is what you want to do. But it isn't a fix for breastfeeding problems, the problem itself needed to be addressed but nobody around me had the tools to do that.

It felt hurtful. My friends and family seemed to want me to turn to formula, thinking it would make me 'happy' again. They didn't realise that breastfeeding had become an all-consuming goal, and if I failed at that, then I felt I failed at everything. Birth had gone badly, this couldn't too. I knew formula could make my life easier in the moment but

I knew it wasn't right for me long term. It was taking a lot of resolve to carry on breastfeeding. I get so tired of the fact that everybody seems so supportive of breastfeeding but the moment something becomes tricky the first response is to turn to formula. It's like a tire blowing on your car and everybody telling you to get the bus.

I can see there are circumstances where breastfeeding can become toxic because I travelled that road a little. It can take away from your joy in motherhood when the experience is so negative. But that doesn't mean 'breastfeeding', as a concept, is wrong. The fault lies with the unsupportive and knowledge-poor society we live in. In my case, it should never have got to this point. Everything I struggled with was avoidable with the right support and information. Had I sought help I could have avoided the heart-ache because I would have rectified my issues with positioning and attachment much earlier.

Lack of support affects far too many women when even a little help could avoid unnecessary suffering. I know some might not breastfeed in the long run but support with that too is just as important. It makes me angry that so many women, who dearly want to breastfeed, are robbed of the experience because they didn't get the support they needed. Women who can (biologically speaking) and want to breastfeed should be enabled to do so, just as those that don't breastfeed should be empowered to formula feed. Feeding a baby is pretty important after all. Support should be there, not only through charities and health professionals, but innate in our society.

I did want a way out. Naturally, I didn't want to dread every feed Fin needed. But I also wanted to feed my baby as

I'd intended. I knew I could get through this somehow.

I searched the internet for ideas of how to get my nipples to heal. After a lot of reading I decided to try to use breast milk itself. It sounded a bit mad at first, but scientifically it made sense given milk's immunological properties.

After each feed, I would express a little milk and gently cover my injuries with it, often also adding a layer of balm. I read that I needed to promote 'moist healing', to stop me from being so scabby.[6] This could only help given how frequently the wound was being pulled about, and I'd already learnt how counter-productive to healing it is (and how much it hurts) when a scab is ripped off.

The breast milk treatment worked wonders. The scabs vanished within a week and nearly all the pain went along with it. It felt like a miracle. Once Finlay was latched on I could feed painlessly for hours if I wanted. Now, with a good latch and healed flesh, I could have cried with relief.

The World Health Organization (WHO) recommends babies are exclusively breastfed for six months and then continue to feed for two years or beyond.[7] I misunderstood the meaning and thought you had to breastfeed for six months and then you could introduce other milks after that if you preferred (perhaps I was falling foul of the marketing of follow-on milks). I'd been steeling myself for six months of pain and I think, had it continued, I may have grinned and bore it, knowing how ridiculously stubborn I can be. My own well-being just didn't register as a priority. Once I realised the recommendation was for two years of breastfeeding, (and beyond!) I was dismayed. I decided to compromise, I would do six months. I'd prepared myself for that already. Any longer just seemed too much to bear, psychologically, at that time.

16

TRYING TIMES

Even with no pain I didn't enjoy breastfeeding. I was glad I'd done it; as a matter of personal success as much as for the benefit of Fin's health. But it wasn't what I had expected. I felt I was doomed to sitting around watching TV, achieving nothing, for the foreseeable future. Fin fed around every hour and a half so I couldn't get anything done or let anybody else look after him. I was a milk factory, and an unwilling one at that.

Since I didn't realise this was biologically normal, and that this stage doesn't last forever, I felt trapped. Nobody had warned me I would be stuck under a baby for months and I wasn't the kind of person to enjoy the rest. People passed comment at how much he fed: 'Oh, he's still hungry,' 'he feeds such a lot,' 'are you sure you have enough milk?' and so on. Since I was insecure about breastfeeding this was all undermining. Instead, I could have done with somebody, laughingly, saying to me, 'Ah, they do feed a lot don't they? Don't worry, it's not forever.'

Fin was a clingy baby and I couldn't put him down

without him screaming like a wounded banshee. These cries cut through me like a knife, with physical pain. I couldn't concentrate on anything else and I would have done *anything* to stop him crying.

I don't believe it's right to leave a baby to cry if you can help it. A baby cries because it needs something. If that's just a cuddle or attention, is it really so bad? It's the only way a small baby can communicate. For a baby who can only see a blurry image of the world it must be frightening to be left alone or put down.

Besides, it's all well and good to say that you should keep putting your baby down so they get used to it, but my little bundle of fury wasn't having any of it. I tried. When I was at my wits end from having held him for hour after hour and day after day, I tried. I put him down and I tried talking to him, sitting with him, giving him things to look at…all to no avail. Although I found it tiresome continually holding Fin, the last thing I wanted was to live with continual screaming. I didn't realise that human babies are born to be carried around, just like other primates, and he would gradually grow in independence. I felt I would be useless forever, eventually holding a grown adult day in, day out.

I didn't recognise that what I was doing was work. Whereas a formula feeding mother has the option (whether she takes it or not) to get some time to herself, it's harder for a breastfeeding mother. You can't ask somebody else to feed the baby whilst you finish what you're doing. You can't pop out for half an hour and ask the person watching the baby to give it a bottle if it gets hungry (unless you express, but that is a whole other story). You have to be on call, all…the…time.

Fortunately, I quickly became adept at managing one-handed, with Finlay in my other arm. Obviously, some things are impossible with one hand: tying your shoelaces, sweeping the floor and cleaning the bath to name a few. But I wanted my independence back. I did what I could.

My saviour came in the form of a baby carrier. I could strap Fin on my front and my hands would be free to get on with *life*. I didn't have to deal with a cumbersome pushchair and, anyway, Fin screamed loudly as soon as I put him in one. Instead, he would fall asleep snuggled against my chest while I got the opportunity to *move*. It helped get him to sleep if he was fussy, too. So, OK, my back ached sometimes, but the benefit to my sanity to be 'up and about' was worth it.

I fed on demand as had been suggested by Ruth (and Fin demanded a lot!). Not having a routine was hard for friends and family to understand. People would lecture me about how he needed to have set sleep times in a specified place and feeding at regular intervals. Apparently I was 'making a rod for my own back'. Supposedly he needed to conform to, what seemed to me, arbitrary social ideals. Fortunately, this was one thing my health visitor was actually supportive of; she agreed he was too little for any routine yet. She suggested it was better to wait and see what Finlay's natural rhythms were and then tailor a routine around that.

Feeding on demand meant we couldn't arrange feeding around a schedule. I was apprehensive about having to breastfeed in front of people; I didn't want to make anyone feel uncomfortable. Feeding around people I didn't know was bad enough, but doing so in front of friends and family somehow seemed worse.

My next essential baby item came as a baby gift sent to me while I was pregnant. Stuart is half American, and his American grandma wanted to send a baby shower gift, it being their tradition. I didn't want a baby shower, even though they're becoming more popular in the UK. I wasn't comfortable with the idea of inviting people round to give me presents. Stuart's grandma, who is endlessly generous, sent a gift anyway. She had emailed to ask if I intended to breastfeed and I replied that I did. I didn't think much more about it. A few weeks later a beautifully wrapped parcel arrived bearing American stamps. It contained lovely baby clothes, swaddling blankets, and a weird piece of black and white patterned fabric. The packaging described it as a breastfeeding cover. It had a strap that went around my neck like an apron, creating a voluminous cloak to hide the baby under. There was a boned section at the top that created a gap so I would be able to see what I was doing.

Although I was grateful, I thought maybe it was an unnecessary accessory and a muslin cloth over the shoulder would do. It transpired that trying to latch on a small baby, who is not good at latching on, when you're not entirely sure what you're doing, and you're feeling embarrassed and flustered, and you can't see because there is a muslin in the way, is not easy. Also babies like to flail about at inopportune moments so that the muslin falls off and exposes your naked breasts.

Initially, the idea of trying to breastfeed in front of people was unthinkable but being covered up gave reassurance.

While I've heard detractors saying these covers perpetuate the idea that breastfeeding should be hidden and that they can draw attention to the person breastfeeding, all I can say is that it made me feel more comfortable.

People were generally fine with me breastfeeding around them. Some friends seemed to find it hard to look me in the eye, but nobody passed comment. Most people paid no attention. Zack sweetly commented to our mum how discreet and chilled I was, although inside I was nervous breastfeeding in front of my big brother.

I was soon sufficiently confident to try breastfeeding in public. Of course, if you take your baby out for longer than, well, half an hour in my case, inevitably your baby will get hungry. So, unless you plan to stay indoors until your baby no longer breastfeeds then this is a hurdle that needs to be got over.

Some women feel driven to hide in toilets to breastfeed but, as well as being unhygienic, I didn't want to sit alone and miss out. I've heard the argument that you should ensure your baby is well fed before you go out and return home before their next feed. I'm afraid breastfeeding doesn't work that way. Besides, it's hard to quantify how much they have eaten and, therefore, how long they can go before they need more. Babies also feed for comfort and, in an unfamiliar setting, they might demand a feed far sooner than they would at home. Sentencing a woman to house arrest for the duration of her breastfeeding life is absurd. Public breastfeeding is a necessity.

My first opportunity came when Fin was a few weeks old. I went shopping with the grandmothers (both our mothers and Stuart's English granny). The hungry cries soon started. My skin prickled with nervous sweat. I spied a bench, and there, like my guardian angel, was another mum feeding her baby! I can't say I'd noticed anyone feeding before, which goes to show how discreet most women are. I was overjoyed; she took the focus off me and provided camaraderie.

I happily sat, swamped my baby in the cover, and got on with it. I'll never forget that woman. If I feel anxious feeding in public I think back to her and remember that I could be giving confidence to a hesitant new mum. Every time you feed outside you're doing something good.

It opened a new world for me. I continued my life but with baby in tow. I felt that, a lot of the time, people didn't realise I had a baby hidden under my cover and, if they did, I knew they couldn't see my breasts. It did wonders for my sanity; being able to leave the house.

When Fin was a month old, we arranged for my lovely nana to meet him for the first time. She lived in a care home and my mum took her out for lunch each week.

We got a table in a corner with nobody around us, for which I was grateful. When Fin began to cry I deftly put on my cover and fed him, continuing to eat and chat. Not for one moment did I consider scurrying off to the car to feed in secret and miss out on this precious time with my nan.

A couple came and sat at the next table and, other than them looking my way a few times, I didn't detect any problem. It was only afterwards my nan said she heard the man complaining the whole time that 'it shouldn't be allowed'. Now, if you have an issue with breastfeeding don't sit on the next table to a woman who is *already breastfeeding*. I was furious, as were the rest of my family. Had we heard him he would have been given a flea in his ear. When we returned to the same restaurant a month or so later I joked with my mum that I hoped the man was there again so I could squirt milk in his eye. *Then* he would have something to complain about!

It infuriates me when people have a negative attitude to public breastfeeding. Fortunately, I rarely came across it. I understand why some people might have an issue with a woman 'flopping her boobs out' (much as I hate the expression) and getting an eyeful. Sure, I can understand that it isn't a regular occurence to see a woman's breasts in public and so this nudity could be disconcerting. But most breastfeeding mums are far from exhibitionists and may be feeling just as embarrassed as you are uncomfortable. Also, the chances are that nobody catches a glimpse of any uncovered skin at all, let alone (God forbid), a nipple.

But then, it is normal to see a woman's breasts on display! Maybe not so much in person, unless people wear very revealing clothes, but on billboards, in magazines, and on TV – sex sells, and breasts sell. So, it's quite all right to see a woman's breasts on display for sexual or commercial reasons, but not if a baby is suckling or if a nipple can be seen. It's quite acceptable for a woman to wear a revealing bikini, but not to reveal a few centimetres of *the same flesh* under a pulled-up, high-necked top?

The vast majority of women feed discretely and it's unlikely anyone else would know what she was doing, let alone catch a glance of skin. But if women don't feel inhibited, if they flash more flesh, then really what is the problem? It's no different to when women are spilling out of low-cut tops; in the great scheme of things, it's just skin. To an extent I agree with discretion. But my use of a cover was for *my* comfort, not others. I see plenty of women who breastfeed without showing any flesh and without using a cover. I also see women who really don't care, and you know what? Good for them. Nipples are only nipples. They're just a slightly different coloured bit of chest. We've all seen them. We all have them. If a woman briefly shows her nipples the world will not stop revolving. Birds will not fall out of the sky. Society will not crumble as hordes of women rip their shirts from their heaving bosoms and race, bare-chested and screaming through the streets.

I jest, but public breastfeeding is a necessity. It helps mothers to engage in everyday life at a tough time in their lives. It exposes others to breastfeeding which, in turn, can be helpful when they have children.[1] Breastfeeding should be part of our consciousness, something we see and something normal. Discreet is one thing (and is a matter of choice), secretive is another.

In general, things were going better. I had largely recovered physically from the birth and was starting to feel more confident with motherhood. I was getting used to, and good at, breastfeeding. My nipples had healed. Life was good!

After dinner one evening I had a sore tummy. I assumed I'd eaten something that didn't agree with me and didn't worry about it. The next day I felt rough again after eating breakfast. It got worse with every meal and soon I found myself with painful stomach cramps and waves of nausea after eating. I would be forced to lie down and, if that coincided with feeding time, then I would have to feed Fin whilst sweating and feeling like I was going to be sick. When you are ill, having a dependent baby is challenging. Again, I was propelled into a situation where breastfeeding was an issue.

Even bland food made me feel rotten. I existed on little more than air. As a breastfeeding mother this was dangerous territory. I needed to eat so the nutrients and calories could be converted into milk. My mystery illness became so bad that, after eating, I was unable even to lift Fin. One night, after perhaps four days, I literally had to lie there while Stuart lifted the baby to my breast to feed. This was not 'just a bug'.

I booked a doctor's appointment, hoping he would give me something to take and I'd be on the mend in a day or two. Mum kindly came to help with Finlay.

'How can I help?' asked my doctor.

'Every time I eat I feel terrible,' I said.

'She's only eating chicken and rice all day. She's breastfeeding a baby, this can't carry on,' my mum interjected. My doctor asked a few questions and then, sighing, started to leaf through a tome of a book.

'You can't take any of these medicines because you're breastfeeding.' He looked at me blankly. 'I'll give you some antacid.'

'So do I have a virus? Is it a bacterial thing?' I asked. Googling my symptoms had left me fretting I could have stomach cancer or an ulcer (googling your symptoms is almost never a good idea).

'Yes, probably,' replied the doctor. I looked at him

perplexed. Clearly, I was getting no more than that. 'You need to eat little and often,' he added.

'But when I eat I can't move…I can't look after my baby. My husband's back at work so I'm home alone,' I argued.

'You need to eat small amounts.' We locked gazes.

'Thank you, doctor,' I said, getting up to leave. I felt, rightly or wrongly, that the doctor was disinterested because he felt my plight was self-induced, in that, if I stopped feeding I could take some medication and recover. Again, I found myself weighing up breastfeeding against my own well-being. What I needed was reassurance that the illness would pass and that Fin wouldn't suffer. Then I would have felt less anxious about riding it out.

It's hard being ill as a new mum. I couldn't crawl away into my bedroom until I got better. I had to look after Fin and be available to feed him. I was up every few hours at night feeding so I didn't get a restorative night's sleep.

Day after day things did not improve. My family was very worried. Stuart, again, tried to stop me from breastfeeding 'for a few days', still not understanding that breastfeeding doesn't work that way. Even if Fin was given my expressed milk for a few days I would still have to express it. I may as well feed it to him directly; cut out the middle man.

Stuart was worried about me and looking for a fix. I promised him that if I lost another half a stone (I had already dropped almost a stone in a week) then I would put Fin on formula and take to my bed.

Inside, I was full of turmoil. Of course, I wanted a rest, but my baby needed feeding and that came first. To breastfeed or not to breastfeed, that was the question.

Other people seemed to think my tenacity was crazy. But, without knowing if I had a tummy bug, stomach cancer or something in between, giving up breastfeeding seemed too reactionary. A few people were concerned that Fin might catch it. I was too, but when I read about it, it seemed that breastfeeding the baby was the best thing I could do. My antibodies would be passed in my milk to the baby to prevent him from catching it, or at least to help him to fight it more easily.

I decided to go back to the doctor.

'I'm not any better. I'm managing with plain food a bit, but I have heartburn now as well,' I told him

'Keep taking the antacid then.'

'It's been nearly two weeks,' I pleaded. 'I can't carry on like this indefinitely.'

'I can't prescribe you any other medication, you're breastfeeding.'

'OK, but, am I going to get better? Is it serious?' I asked.

'You will get better,' he replied. You would expect a health professional to be concerned at the drain the illness was having on a nursing mother. You would think that some care or compassion would be in order. Clearly not!

Fortunately, after this visit my health began to turn around of its own accord, just in time for me not to quit breastfeeding. I'd been trying bits of other foods periodically and now I found my body would tolerate vegetables other than peas and meat other than chicken. Eating a baked potato was sensational. It seemed I wasn't going to die and I could carry on breastfeeding. Two victories!

The following week the health visitor came to do Fin's

six week check. I told her about how ill I'd been. 'Oh yes, that's nasty, it's been going around lately. Takes a few weeks to get over, doesn't it?' she said. I stared at her dumbfounded. All that worry and it was just a bug that had been doing the rounds! I'd spent two weeks convincing myself I had a serious disease. I had argued with my closest friends and family about whether I needed to stop breastfeeding or not; arguing when I was ill and looking after a tiny baby. All of this could have been avoided had I known it was a nasty bug that would go. Surely, the doctor must have come across it too? I was furious. Again my breastfeeding journey had been threatened by lack of support and with the only suggestion for remedy being to stop.

At the same health visitor appointment I was also checked for postnatal depression. I had to fill in a questionnaire as a basis for this assessment. It featured questions along the lines of:

'In the past week I have felt sad...

a) most of the time

b) quite often

c) not very often

d) not at all.'

Now, I'm not a psychiatrist, but I don't think it's hard to figure out how to fiddle the system if you don't want people to know you feel down. Nonetheless, I decided to be honest. It didn't come out well. I'd been through a lot. I wasn't diagnosed with postnatal depression on the basis that my misery was circumstantial, the health visitor simply wanted to see me again sooner than usual. But considering how I felt I didn't appreciate the next exchange.

'So have you had any smiles yet?' she asked.

'No, not that aren't wind,' I said.

'Hmm…well he should be smiling. It's probably because you've been so unhappy. You haven't been smiling enough so he isn't smiling back.' She delivered this damning news with seemingly no realisation that it was a knife in my sore heart.

I was hindering my baby's progress because I was too sad. I suppose I should grin at him like a buffoon even when I was dying inside. The truth may be that his development in this area was just slow. These things are variable after all. But I was made to feel that I had done something wrong. Anyway, I did smile at him and, of course, I wasn't the only face he saw. Besides, how do you think blind people learn to smile? What a terrible thing to suggest to somebody who was clearly struggling, that I had stunted my baby's development by being down.

In retrospect, perhaps I wasn't just sad. Is it depression if you are feeling wretched because life is hard? Should it not still mean that you get an offer of support? Those days seem dark and…lost. Every time I started to claw my way out of the hole I was shoved back down.

It makes me so angry that it was induced by thoughtless postnatal care and support. Looking back now at the bleakness of those days I think I could have done with something. Not medication, but perhaps a chat with someone. Just because I had good reason to be down doesn't seem a good reason not to follow it up (it wasn't followed up; I was asked if I was feeling all right a few weeks later, to which I replied that I was fine). It's not even as if my returning health heralded a new-found joy and optimism. As

I look back, the months that followed were plagued with lingering anxiety and paranoia.

At four months Fin would cry continually unless he was latched to a breast. An internet search told me to just go with it, since it's a normal developmental phase.[2] I made sure I had some good telly to watch, and prepared to sit and feed a lot until it was over. It worked like a dream and we were soon back on track.

My body had risen to the challenge of meeting his changing needs. I should have given myself credit; I was breastfeeding successfully, even if I did have to seek out solutions to problems myself on the internet. Really, I'd come such a long way.

My health was returned; my baby was a picture of health and happiness (and could now smile); and breastfeeding seemed to be under control. I was out and about, going to baby groups, meeting friends, strapping Fin into a carrier and tramping round the countryside. I had even started going jogging (when I could escape) in an effort to get my body back.

The sad fact remained that I still didn't *like* breastfeeding. I was impressed by all the positive aspects of feeding and it was amazing seeing my baby grow as a result of food I was physically producing. Biologically speaking, I found the process fascinating. However, I found it tiresome, boring and restrictive. I also found the interrupted nights insanity-inducing. I hadn't expected it all to be so *hard.*

I would feed until six months and not a day longer. I had a fantasy that when Finlay was six months old I would hand

Stuart a bottle of formula, book into a hotel for the night and refuse to tell anyone where I was. I would sleep and sleep and sleep; not having to be available for milk or jump the instant I heard crying.

My days of breastfeeding were numbered and I was glad.

17

BABIES AND BEDS

Historically, as still happens today in tribal communities, babies slept with their mothers; in her arms or by her side.[1] In fact, babies would be found with their mothers all the time; our young expect to be carried, feeding at will.

Bed-sharing is common practice in many developing countries, but in Europe and America it's often frowned upon. Not only are babies carried less in the day, but they are expected to sleep alone, in a separate cot, and even a separate room, during the night.

Since the eighteenth century the idea of babies needing to sleep independently has proliferated.[2(pp51-76)] Prior to this, families would have shared a room. In fact, my grandmother, in the early 1900s, grew up in a two-room cowshed, where her parents slept in one room with the littlest ones as necessary, whilst she and up to thirteen of her other siblings shared the other. That's perhaps an extreme example of rural Irish living, but my point is that this is not ancient history, and yet the idea of living in such close quarters is now unthinkable. Sharing beds, particularly with babies, is horrifying to many. Stories abound in the press of babies who have died whilst asleep with their parents, having suffocated, or died for unexplained reasons. You can understand why people don't like the idea.

But yet, our animal instincts drive us to sleep together. Babies seem to sleep more contentedly and breastfeeding is easier.[3] That breastfeeding hormone, oxytocin, makes you feel drowsy too.[2(p143)] So, when a mother wakes up, tired, to feed her baby the feeling is compounded by the hormones she releases. It's natural to doze off to sleep with your baby.

If a baby is sleeping alone, when they wake their caregiver needs to get out of bed and help them get back to sleep, perhaps by feeding them. This in itself can take a long time, so sleep is not only interrupted, but interrupted for a long period. By this point you will have woken more fully and it can be harder to get back to sleep. In order to cope with that, methods have evolved to 'train' the baby to sleep.

Some methods focus on 'extinction' techniques.[4] Here, the baby is left to cry for increasing amounts of time (so you might soothe them after one minute, then two, then three, and so on). The baby 'learns' to settle themselves without a parent. These methods are sometimes also called 'controlled crying' or 'cry it out'.

Other, gentler, techniques focus on building routines so that babies learn to respond to cues to tell them when it's time to settle down to sleep.[5] There will be a night-time routine to signal that it's bedtime, perhaps with a bath and a story. Sometimes gentle music might be used. The baby might have a particular toy that they find comforting or they might use a dummy. The parents will also think about how the day is structured to ensure that the baby is ready to sleep, that it won't be wide awake or, equally disruptive, over-tired.

Even though sleep training is commonplace and bed-sharing largely frowned upon, it's estimated that around half of UK mums share a bed with their baby at some point.[6] So, whatever your opinion on where a baby should sleep, it's important to address how to sleep safely with a baby. It's considerably safer to think about the possibility of bed-sharing and ensure the family bed is a safe place, than to fall asleep by accident in a potentially dangerous environment such as a sofa where a baby could get wedged between cushions or be dropped.[7] It's important to be up to date with recommendations concerning infant sleep.

Research into safe sleep is ongoing. Current recommendations in the UK are for babies to sleep in their own cots in their parents' room[8] since this seems to be the safest set-up. However, statistics around bed-sharing can be muddied by the inclusion of data of when bed-sharing has been unintentional, so, for instance, when sharing a sofa with a baby or when being under the influence of drugs.

However, when making a decision about where a baby sleeps, it's important to look at the bigger picture. Although breastfed babies have been found to not disrupt sleep more than formula-fed babies,[9] when they do wake the burden falls on one person. If the breastfeeding mother is woken regularly, every night, for weeks (fighting the hormones that make her drowsy) then she's going to be tired. That then has implications for the daytime such as whether she can drive a car safely or whether she might accidentally fall asleep with the baby somewhere unsafe because she's exhausted. Sometimes, looking at the big picture, I think bed-sharing can be the safer option. Given that most parents sleep with their babies at one time or another, if we don't inform parents on safe co-sleeping then unplanned co-sleeping becomes dangerous. Rather than a blanket message not to do it, the 'experts' ought to provide guidelines on how to do it safely.

Of course, in some circumstances it's *not* safe. It's unsafe to bed-share if you're excessively tired, are on medication, have been drinking, smoking or taking drugs, nor is it safe to sleep on a sofa or if the baby is swaddled.[10] Bed-sharing may also be riskier for formula feeding mothers due to the way they position themselves with the baby in the bed.[11]

It's imperative to consider the safety of the adult bed, and to consider the issue of your baby falling out. Some people sleep at floor level (for instance, on a mattress). Others use co-sleeping cribs or bed guards. It's also important to consider that adult bedclothes, such as duvets and pillows, are unsafe near a baby, so they need to be kept away or removed.[12] Provided that we're well informed of what is dangerous then we can make the best choices for our circumstances and environment.

We all want our babies to be safe. But we need to understand what's normal for babies and how that can be dealt with. We have a cultural notion that babies should sleep in a cot, possibly in a nursery, and that by a certain number of weeks they should be sleeping through the night. The truth is that some children don't sleep through the night for months, or even years.[13] It seems to me that, rather than struggling against the 'problem', we ought to be looking at ways to cope with what's normal.

If families choose for their baby to sleep in a separate

bed or in a separate room then coping mechanisms during the day are even more important. It's often suggested that women should try to sleep when their babies do, the housework can wait. Getting other people to pick up the pieces for you, or to help care for the baby while you sleep, is also useful. Caring for young babies is hard and our communities make a big difference to how well we cope.

It's up to individual families to choose where their babies sleep, as long as that place is as safe as possible when you look at the bigger picture of your parenting situation. If a mother chooses for her baby to sleep in a cot because she feels it's the safer option, she doesn't sleep well with her baby, she feels her baby sleeps better or whatever reason then that's up to her. If the mum and baby sleep together but the dad decides to sleep elsewhere because the baby disrupts his sleep then that's up to them. It's about equipping people with the information and tools so what they do fits their own families as well as being safe.

Oh, and as a side note, if you think that sleeping with a baby prohibits a sex life then you have no imagination. Sex doesn't always have to take place in the marital bed at a set time. Where there's a will, there's a way.

We need to be honest that breastfeeding at night is a tough job. The solution isn't to remove breastfeeding from the equation, by formula feeding or expressing milk, or to use harsh sleep training methods, it's to look at our biological roots and how women have coped with the situation for millennia. In my opinion, fixing our sleeping arrangements is more important than 'fixing' the babies themselves.

18

SLEEP, OR LACK THEREOF

Although everybody tells you to catch up on sleep before you have your baby, I'd found this virtually impossible. Initially, my painful breasts made it difficult to get comfortable. Then I started to need cushions and pillows to prop up my growing bump. Every night I would lie sleepless and angry.

In hospital Fin slept well, only waking occasionally and making little sucking and squeaking noises for a feed. Unfortunately, I didn't get the same pleasure. Besides lovingly gazing at his face, I was kept awake by the constant stream of doctors and nurses and when one baby stopped crying another started up. Sleep wasn't going to happen.

At home Fin slept beautifully in his Moses basket beside me for two nights. Around every two or three hours I was woken by his searching noises and I propped myself up in bed and fed him. Once he was fast asleep again I popped him back in his Moses basket where he slept soundly until the next feed. Through the day we followed a similar pattern, except that some of his sleeping was done in people's arms.

This was amazing! I could survive on this routine. I never expected it to be so easy. These silly women complaining about getting no sleep with a newborn. It was all so simple!

Then day three arrived. For absolutely no reason, Finlay decided he didn't like sleeping in his own bed and would instantly wake and scream his little head off if he was moved from my arms.

We tried *everything*. I fed him, we rocked him, we cuddled him, we sang to him, we changed his nappy and we winded him. I couldn't understand it. He would be zonked out in a milk-fuelled snooze, but the second I placed him into his bed he would start screaming again. At stupid o'clock in the morning, with us both staring, bewildered at this furious newborn, a sudden brain-wave made me fetch a swaddling blanket that Laura had bought us. This was the type that's pre-shaped so you just Velcro it around the baby's arms, rather than needing lots of tucking and folding that I wouldn't have been able to figure out when befuddled from sleeplessness. We stuffed Fin in this little straight-jacket and he fell instantly asleep. We were victorious!

It never worked again. At the next wake-up call, when we had tried everything we could think of, Stuart said, 'Why don't you bring him in with us?' I felt guilty about 'giving up' but, having not slept properly for weeks and still recovering from labour, I did exactly that. I fed Fin till he fell asleep and then snuggled up and joined him.

This may seem uncharacteristically weak-willed of me, that after one rough night I gave up and took my baby to bed. At one time, I would have considered this to be too dangerous. Babies sleep in cots in their own rooms and if they come into bed with you, you will roll on them and kill them, right?

A friend of mine, Ben, had told me the story of when his children were tiny. When his firstborn came along, he and his wife got rid of their bed frame and slept on their mattress on the floor with the baby. When number two arrived, child number one graduated to his own floor mattress and number two took his place on his parents' mattress. I had smiled and nodded while privately thinking this was a family of hippy weirdos. But when I fell pregnant, Ben bought me a book about bed-sharing called *Three in a Bed* by Deborah Jackson.[1] He explained that, when they had been having trouble getting their eldest son to sleep, he'd bought the book for his wife and it had led to their floor mattresses. I still thought they were nuts, but I'll read anything.

Actually, I read every pregnancy book I could find. They all seemed to offer similar advice. There was a formula to getting a baby that behaved like clockwork. Baby had to go to bed, in a cot, while drowsy but not asleep. He should be left to cry for short periods. He would then learn to get himself off to sleep. If he woke 'too soon' after a feed he shouldn't get any more milk. He had to have a dark, quiet room, but not too quiet or he would be disturbed by every sound. The list was endless. It troubled me that there was no flexibility. Surely, all babies were not alike? If it worked, why did people complain about the difficulties of infant sleep? Finlay didn't appear to want to sleep alone, in a cot, in a dark, quiet room for periods of three to four hours. He wanted to sleep in my arms and feed every one to two hours. Not feeding him back to sleep was unthinkable, unless you like the continual noise of a crying baby. It was the easiest way to get him to sleep.

Thank goodness for *Three in a Bed*. Initially, I was horrified. These lazy parents were sharing their beds because they couldn't be bothered to make the effort to teach their babies to sleep in the *right* place (bear in mind I was pregnant when I read it, so hadn't yet learned that babies don't seem to cooperate much with 'teaching'). But, as I read on, I began to be persuaded by the arguments for bed-sharing; in its normality and safety. Moreover, I felt freed from the 'formula' of infant care.

To illustrate, here's one of my favourite excerpts from the book:

The 'idea' of carrying and sleeping with your baby is not intended to create in parents a state of nervous guilt. I've presented my research, now I am letting you off the hook. Don't be frightened to put your baby down. Don't sleep with your baby if you don't want to. The title of the book is a concept, not a prescription. If you find some ideas which appeal, use them to inform your actions, rather than to overwhelm them. Sleep with your baby because it's fun and it suits you. Carry him because it gives you pleasure, not because I tell you to. You'll learn far more from the baby than from me, and maybe some of his natural confidence will rub off.[1(p253)]

I realised I didn't need a plan. I could just follow Fin's lead.

I also became aware that I might have to seek out alternative parenting ideas amongst the plethora of conventional literature.

It made sense to me, biologically, to bed-share, but I decided to keep my options open; I was still apprehensive given a lifetime of social conditioning to cots.

That third night, when my inconsolable son wanted to be in my arms, I broke willingly. Bed-sharing was always going to be more my style than leaving a baby in a cot to cry. When Fin cried, every instinct I had pushed me towards holding him and catering to his every need, not leaving him alone, even with regular check-ins to pat him. Instinctively, I knew that my immature baby needed me; to feel my warmth and hear my heartbeat.

If Fin wouldn't stay asleep in a cot then what else was I to do anyway? I couldn't very well stay up all night, every night. Crying it out (in its various forms) might work for other people, but in my heart it felt cruel. There's a lot of sleep 'advice' out there, but there's one thing that's pretty much guaranteed to get a baby back to sleep and that's feeding it.

If you add into the mix that Fin woke every hour and a half to feed, bed-sharing was the only way I could cope. If I got up and fed Fin in a rocking chair, potentially for an hour, every hour and a half, well...I don't like that kind of maths. Bed-sharing meant I could feed and sleep at the same time, which saved my sanity, preserved my breastfeeding relationship (because I wasn't tempted to get somebody else to give him a bottle so I could sleep), and stopped me falling asleep accidentally. Had I not been made aware of the option of taking my baby to bed, my parenting journey would have looked very different. I can assure you that breastfeeding wouldn't have lasted. Now, I suppose I've joined the ranks of 'hippy weirdos,' and thank goodness I did.

Nonetheless, bed-sharing is a contentious subject and you should always do what you think is safe and right. I was still nervous of over-laying and suffocating my baby. Although, Ben made a good point: 'You don't roll all over your husband while you sleep, do you?' I can't fault that logic. It's not like I fall out of bed every night, unaware I was near the edge. When you're asleep you still know where you are. I came to the conclusion that, provided I was alert (as in, not having taken medication and so on), I was likely to know exactly where my baby was during the night.

I would go to sleep in the recovery position so I couldn't roll, with my arms encircling and protecting Fin, tucking the covers firmly around my legs so they couldn't possibly go near him. We attached Fin's cot to our bed, ensuring there were no gaps around the mattresses (we didn't buy a co-sleeper cot because they weren't so commonplace then). It meant he was in no danger of falling off the edge of the bed and he had his own space in the cot if I managed to push him away from me. Thanks to breastfeeding, Fin would be at my bust level and nowhere near my pillows. When he woke for a feed I only needed to rouse for mere seconds to latch him on. I was probably one of the best-rested new mums you could ever meet; my awakenings were short and drowsy.

The alternative was, in my humble opinion, a nightmare. You feed the baby for an hour, you struggle to get them to go down in their cot and then an hour or two later you're up again repeating the process. Yes, it's possible to do this for a few days but for *months*? By having Fin in my bed I could function the next day. I could look after him, go to groups, do housework, drive safely, and feed him without falling asleep in a chair or dropping him.

In an ideal world, Fin would have slept wherever it was safest, which at the time was considered to be in a cot in our room. But I also had to consider the safety of his being in my care if I was chronically sleep deprived, as well as my psychological well-being. On balance, bed-sharing was, for me, the safest answer.

My mum (amongst others) told me that 'in her day' if your baby woke a lot you crumbled a rusk in their bottle before bed, but, unless I scattered them on my breasts I didn't see how it would work. A bottle of formula before bed was mooted by many. As with any breastfeeding-related difficulty, formula is so often seen as the answer. To me, the response to him digesting my milk fast was not to give him something harder to digest. I didn't want to introduce a bottle at bedtime because of the possible effect on my milk supply. I had to work with the reality of exclusive breastfeeding and what that meant for sleep.

Fin didn't even like sleeping in other people's arms and, of course, nobody else got to feed him either. I felt guilty for feeding him 'too often' and for cuddling him 'too much'. I felt judged so I would apologise when he needed to feed, as though I were doing something wrong, especially when people asked if he was hungry *again*. But, for now, this little primitive baby needed his mum.

I did love sleeping with my little boy (when I didn't feel guilty). It was a wonderful experience. I was never woken by crying, only by fidgeting indicating that he was hungry. He used to make a noise like he was clearing his throat, as if to say: 'Ahem, Mummy! Milk please!' While I was still getting over the labour it was great not to have to keep getting him in and out of a cot. I had sufficient sleep and I could recover.

It was amazing how aware of Finlay I was. I would wake up stiff from having not moved a muscle in the night. Stuart once told me he'd watched me soothing Fin back to sleep without so much as opening my eyes. I could respond to him in my sleep!

I didn't mention this sleeping arrangement to my health visitor for fear of criticism. She'd made it clear by her suggestions about sleep ('make sure he goes in his cot when he's drowsy, not asleep,' and so on), that she was unlikely to approve.

I remember one health visitor coming over and asking how he was sleeping. I told her (without letting on that he slept in my bed) that he woke up about five times a night and that, yes, I was tired. Regular waking, even if short, is still tiring. You still don't get into a deep, restorative sleep. She proceeded to lecture me on self-soothing. It felt like a broken record.

Why could nobody see there were alternatives? I didn't have to leave Fin to cry in order to learn to sleep. I was a parent twenty-four hours a day; I shouldn't refuse to deal with him 'out-of-hours'. It was also perfectly natural to feed him to sleep, I wasn't teaching him bad habits, I was getting him to sleep in the way that mothers have for millennia.

I meekly said I would give it a go (keeping my fingers crossed behind my back). This is when I started to practice appeasement with certain health professionals. I understood they had to give an approved line of advice and I decided that if I didn't agree with it I wasn't about to get into an argument. After all, it wasn't going to change my mulish mind.

I had been fairly open with my family about how we slept, but they too started to lecture me about 'letting him have a little cry'. So, I told them that we no longer bed-shared. I didn't need any additional pressure on top of what I already put myself under.

In the evenings of those early weeks, Fin would sleep in my arms until Stuart and I decided to go to bed. It was nice to have baby cuddles, although the weight and heat of the baby, and my inability to move for fear of disturbing him, did get frustrating. Once our bedtime arrived I would gently carry Fin up to bed and lay him next to me where he would sleep all night, feeding when he wanted.

Still, I longed for a little time to myself, an evening would do. I knew it might be a frustrating process to start to settle him in his cot so I picked a few days that I could dedicate to it. I waited until Stuart was working evenings for a few days and I took the opportunity to 'play' with settling Fin.

I had already initiated a bedtime routine; bath, story and bed. So once the 'bed' phase started, instead of heading downstairs to spend my evening with Stuart, I got my pyjamas on and prepared to spend the evening in our bedroom. I got my laptop, and a stack of books and magazines so I could sit all evening trying different things without getting bored.

Initially, Fin would wake instantly when I put him down after a feed (as he had done since he was three days old). Even if I slowly moved away by millimetres, my arms burning and my hands going to sleep, he would still wake up. If he stirred I could sometimes soothe him back to sleep by letting him suck on my fingers like he would a dummy, but failing that, I would have to go back to feeding him again.

Eventually, I perfected putting Fin down gently, but he didn't stay asleep for long. Having a big feed did help but, after further trial and error, I found that swaddling him seemed to increase the amount of time he slept (of course, when I came to bed I would remove his swaddles for safety). This was progress. When Stuart's shift changed again, and he was at home in the evenings, I was able to sit with him without Fin.

While Fin slept in our bed for a portion of every night, Stuart was anxious about the arrangement. I too felt the pressure to get Fin to sleep in his own bed consistently. At each feed I would try to settle him in his own room until I got to a point where I couldn't bear it any longer and brought him into bed with us. It wasn't laziness; I was exhausted. I hoped for the night when I could put him in his cot and for him to stay there, asleep, until morning.

As Fin got older, and I suppose as he got used to it, he slept for slightly longer stretches. The first time he managed a two hour stretch I was in a state of panic, worrying he was dead, rather than asleep. I kept going to check, each time risking waking him up. I watched, holding my breath and watching for the rise and fall of his chest; this couldn't be Fin, sleeping alone? But it was.

Still, once I got to the small hours of the morning, despite the longer stretches of sleep, I would still bring Fin into our bed so that I could get a patch of less-interrupted sleep. In the day, I let him sleep in my arms or in his cot depending on what I was up to. At least this way I could settle Fin into his cot. I had options.

I didn't want to use a dummy. I felt they were dirty and ugly. I had also read that dummy use can impact on breastfeeding due to the baby not stimulating milk production by suckling. I worried, too, that it might affect our newly improved latch. Then there was the question of how, in the long term, we would get a dummy off Fin. I didn't want him to be a toddler who always had a dummy in his mouth. On the other hand, dummies reduce the risk of SIDS (Sudden Infant Death Syndrome)[2] and could help with settling him during those long, interrupted nights.

Stuart was keen to try dummies. He'd seen how tired I was and obviously had been worried about me when I was so ill. He thought a dummy could help. If Fin would go back to sleep sucking a finger, surely he would sleep with a dummy (and my finger wouldn't get so pruney)? Stuart saw dummies as nothing more than a useful tool.

Stuart deserved to have some input in our parenting decisions. Up until this point, I'd called the shots for most things. Our families were in agreement that a dummy would help. Eventually, I caved in on this one little thing.

I'd been toying with my decision when I had to take Fin to hospital for a blood test because, at six weeks, he was still jaundiced. Although he was only tinged yellow by this point, my health visitor wanted to send us to check that the bilirubin levels in his blood were safe. Looking back now, I wonder if this ongoing jaundice was a sign that breastfeeding hadn't been going so well,[3(p84)] but it seemed nobody made this connection.

There was a drop in clinic at the hospital where Fin had been born so this blood test promised to be quick. Stuart was sleeping off a night shift so I went alone.

On arrival I received a frosty welcome, with them completely flummoxed as to why I had 'just turned up'.

'The health visitor said to come. She said she would phone?' I said. The nurse on reception looked doubtful.

'OK, go to the waiting room. Someone will be with you shortly,' she said.

Hours passed. While I waited, a particular nurse (I shall call her Friendly Nurse) kindly offered me a room to breastfeed in, but I declined, I was happy breastfeeding in the waiting room of a paediatric ward.

Eventually, a doctor called Finlay's name and the nurse escorted me into a small office attached to the triage ward. She started sorting paperwork and then disappeared, seemingly to get something. While I waited, I read the posters, I walked around soothing Fin, I nosed at the shelves of syringes and bandages and marvelled at how they were mislabelled.

Getting bored, I looked for Friendly Nurse and asked her where my doctor had gone. She clearly located her, because the doctor came bustling back in, seemingly much too busy to be troubled with us. She hooked Fin up to a heart monitor and he started to whinge. His heartbeat soared as his cries became more piercing. I put a finger into his mouth for him to suck and I immediately noticed his heartbeat plummet. To me this was proof that sucking was calming. This was what gave me the final push to use a dummy; I could see the physical response. It wasn't just acting as a cork, stopping him from crying, it was helping him feel better.

The blood test was horrid. A nurse held Fin still while the doctor took his blood. I was instructed to drip glucose solution into his mouth from a syringe. Fin seemed to be torn between loving the sugar and hating the pain of the procedure. It was, at least, over quickly.

I thought I'd be allowed to go home to await the test results, but the doctor wanted me to wait until they were processed. I was allowed to leave the site to get myself some lunch as we had come completely unprepared and I was starving. Thank goodness I was breastfeeding or I would have run out of milk.

When I returned for the results, Friendly Nurse went to find them. Time passed. Tumbleweed rolled by. Friendly Nurse, finally, seemed to pin down a doctor who was ushered in looking harassed. He informed me that the tests were perfectly fine, but I had to wait for them to write up the paperwork before I could go home. Seriously annoyed, I returned to the same ugly, old sofa in the waiting room. Friendly Nurse happened to walk past and looked horrified,

'Why are you *still* here?' she asked.

'The doctor said I had to wait for him to write up the paperwork,' I replied, shrugging.

'You are joking!' she cried. 'You've been here too long

already. I'll personally make sure the paperwork gets posted to you. Go home!'

'Are you sure?' I asked, worried that I should wait.

'Of course, go!' After eight and a half hours for a minor blood test, I finally left.

When I got home I was in tears. I'd been kept in an infectious environment with a tiny baby and I was exhausted. I know there were seriously ill children there and, naturally, they needed to be prioritised, but a whole day's wait was too much.

This was the same hospital where I'd cried, alone, after a long and traumatising labour. This was where I had received not so much as a paracetamol, let alone *care* following Fin's birth. I'd been forgotten on both of my visits there.

I needed to do something productive, to ensure they realised that what I had endured was *wrong*. I poured my vitriol into a three page, cathartic, letter; straight to the chief of the hospital. A few weeks later I received a letter of apology. Vindicated, I moved on with my life.

Anyway, I thought I ought to at least give dummies a try. I wanted to be the one to choose which ones we would use so I still retained a certain amount of control. I went to the supermarket and chose some expensive, orthodontic dummies. They were clear plastic so I could still see Fin's little face and they offended me less.

I went home and confessed my purchase to Stuart. I hadn't yet told him about my change of heart. He sterilised them right away, having won a rare victory. I gently, apprehensively, placed a dummy into Finlay's mouth. He pulled a face and the dummy sailed across the room. I tried tapping it with a fingernail as I'd seen some mums do. It still got spat out. I tried putting a bit of expressed milk on it. Still no. Nothing worked. Now that I'd decided to try I was determined to get it to work.

One of our friends told us that their babies preferred the cheaper kinds of dummy. I read that some babies prefer latex dummies because they're softer (although there is an allergy risk). I also heard that you should look for types that are similar in size to your own nipples. We soon amassed a collection of all different kinds each of which Fin rejected, some more forcefully than others.

When we did manage to persuade Fin to take a dummy and suck it until he fell asleep, as he relaxed it would fall out of his mouth. This meant that if he woke up he wouldn't be able to settle back to sleep. Using a dummy didn't really achieve what we wanted.

However, dummies were useful for the car. I was getting tired of spending every journey listening to Fin cry. He got particularly upset if the car stopped moving so I would go to great lengths not to stop. I often had to play 'do a whole journey without stopping'. It's fun and annoys other road users. Anyway, dummies helped to keep me from being distracted by him while I was driving, but that was largely all I used them for.

I'd never realised what real tiredness was. I struggled to have any enthusiasm for anything and I had a lower attention span than a fish. I would get so annoyed at other (childless) people telling me they were tired from one late night. My eyes were panda ringed and my face was haggard. I thought that this was now my face, for perpetuity.

Of course, simultaneously, everybody I met would be asking how Fin was sleeping. Even strangers will ask that as one of the first questions, 'Is he a good baby, does he sleep?' Eyebrows would be raised about his frequency of waking even though, in reality, it was normal for such a young baby.

I continued to ride out the storm. Weaning on to solids came and went and made no difference. I read *The No-Cry Sleep Solution* by Elizabeth Pantley[4] to try some gentle sleep training but I only used a few tips, such as considering the last hour before bedtime and the pattern of his daytime sleep. Following a suggestion in the book, I bought a noise-activated, music generator so as soon as Fin stirred it would play soothing music or sounds. It only helped in masking the sound of me leaving the room. Each thing that offered us hope had such a small impact and turned excitement into disappointment.

Gradually, Fin started to improve, but it was slow; two steps forwards and one step back. Every night I would wonder, optimistically, whether tonight would be the night when he would sleep through whilst I also had an internal dread that it would be *another* sleepless night. The only reason I managed to get any sleep in this mood was because I was so exhausted. I would pass out as soon as my head hit the pillow.

At night I started to get frustrated that often, just as I went to bed, as soon as I got drowsy and warm, Fin would cry and I would have to rouse myself and feed him. To tackle this I tried giving him a 'dream feed'. I would go upstairs before I was planning to go to bed, pick Fin up gently and feed him with only the minimal amount of waking. When I then went to bed I would get an hour or two of sleep before the next feed. I hoped that, eventually, he might stop waking for that feed as he was used to snoozing through it.

When Fin was around seven months we were, again, struggling. It coincided with me trying to wean him off swaddling because, now that he was moving more, he could easily get himself tangled up. I should have got rid of the swaddles long before, but they made him sleep so much better. He also started to show signs of teething. The two combined added up to a lot of waking up.

I was, yet again, reaching the end of my endurance and doubting my night-time parenting decisions. I went to a local baby group one week and was talking about it to the other mums. They *all* had babies who slept through the night. Although, for the most part, I was envious of them there was a weird sort of pride that my baby was a bit different; *I* had the baby that didn't sleep.

Anyway, the lady who ran the group joined the conversation.

'There was a lady who used to come here,' she told us, 'and she had the same thing. It's funny; she always looked fresh as a daisy. You'd never believe she didn't get any sleep. One time she came along completely haggard. We all wondered what the matter was. Turns out, it was the first time her baby had actually slept!' We all laughed.

'Actually, I have something for you,' she said, looking at me. I followed her to her bag. She pulled out some sheets and pressed them into my hand. 'This might help you to sort things out.'

'Thanks, I'll take a look,' I replied. I liked this lady, she often had useful things to say, so I thought I'd have a read. In the car I eagerly scanned the sheets, to find it was yet another guide to controlled crying. She had clearly never listened to a word I said about my preference for gentle parenting. Everybody was telling me this was the solution but my heart told me that it couldn't be right.

Fin's sleep improved anyway. Then, out of nowhere, when I was feeling around his swollen little gums there was a little, sharp, hard patch. There it was; the first tooth! It had erupted without a fuss.

When Fin had first shown signs of teething I'd looked into the consequences for breastfeeding. Teeth didn't seem like a positive development. I'd heard people say they wouldn't breastfeed a baby with teeth and I could understand the worry. Still, the information I'd read said teeth don't stop breastfeeding as it's the tongue, not the gums or teeth, which extracts the milk.[2(p123)] So far this appeared to be right, I couldn't tell there was anything different. I hadn't been sure how people continued to breastfeed long term unless they had Kevlar nipples; it turns out that teeth don't matter.

One night, when Fin was about ten months old, I went to bed after the dream feed as normal, prepared for the worst. When I woke up, I jumped up in shock because it was light outside and there was no baby in my bed. My gasp woke Stuart who was also confused. I blearily looked at the clock. It was six o'clock! I'd got seven hours sleep for the first time in living memory; or so it seemed. I darted out of bed panic-stricken that Fin was dead but at his door I could hear him snoring. I smiled.

So much sleep! I didn't expect for a minute that my good luck would continue, but it did. I even dropped the dream feed and was amazed to find that I had a baby who slept through the night. In retrospect, I was lucky that this happened before he was one but, at the time, it seemed I'd waited an age as he went from waking five times a night to not waking at all.

Lack of sleep for one night is hard, but for months? I thought I was losing my mind. It's especially hard when that goes hand-in-hand with the upheaval and emotion of being a first-time parent. So many of my friends seemed to have babies that slept and their solution was that they formula-fed and used controlled crying. It made me feel like I was doing it wrong, that my mothering instincts were wrong. It made me wonder whether maybe breast milk wasn't enough.

It took a lot to stop fighting my paranoia and realise that what I was doing wasn't 'wrong', it was just unusual in my peer circle. I wasn't surrounded with fellow zombies who could reassure me and give me tips. Bed-sharing and feeding to sleep was about survival and, at the time, I didn't know anybody else who lived this way.

I felt proud that I'd managed to muddle along and come out of the other side reasonably unscathed. Along the way I got to hold Finlay while he slept, something that I wistfully remember now. I was the person he linked with food, sleep and comfort and he would instantly calm down when he saw me. I managed to resist the temptation (and social pressure) to give formula or leave him to cry in the hope of more sleep that probably wouldn't have happened anyway. Whatever the arguments might be, I'd do it all again, sleepless nights and all.

19

WHY BOTHER BREASTFEEDING?

I've probably not made breastfeeding sound all that appealing up to now. It was tough in those early days, and during those difficult moments it was hard to keep sight of why I was bothering. But, I promise, the good times have made it completely worthwhile. Still, it was good to know, when I was struggling, that there was a point to all this.

I think most people's decision to breastfeed would be based on the personal benefit to them and their baby. Breastfeeding is the biological norm for feeding human babies. Both mothers' and babies' bodies are designed to function this way. As in so many things, diverting from the natural course of things can bring a whole raft of issues.

In unhygienic situations the decision to formula feed can mean life or death. If formula milk is prepared in unclean conditions, or if it's watered down to make it last longer, then it's not a safe food for babies. Although this may seem extreme 'in this day and age' it's still a problem, including in refugee camps where people are fleeing war-torn countries.[1] In developed nations, however, formula is seen as a safe alternative. While that's true to an extent, breastfeeding is still the way our bodies are designed to be fed.

Nutritionally, breast milk is bespoke, meeting the changing needs of the baby. As I've already said, the nutrients will be perfectly tailored to your baby's needs and the antibodies support the baby's maturing immune system. Since the mother is exposed to the same pathogens as that of the baby, she will produce the perfect antibodies to pass on to protect her child. Unsurprisingly, breastfed babies are less at risk of infections.[2] Benefits last into adulthood, with studies showing reduced risks of obesity,[3] diabetes[4] and some cancers.[5] Since breastfeeding also helps to establish the gut microbiome there may also be far-reaching consequences such as reduced risk of allergies.[6]

It's not a one-way thing. Mothers also benefit from breastfeeding. It lowers the risk of some cancers (including breast cancer)[7] and cardiovascular disease.[8] Breastfeeding helps mothers to regain their figures after having a baby and delays the return of periods.[7] It even has a contraceptive effect.[9]

Breastfeeding, once it's established, is really convenient. You don't need to remember to buy milk or prepare bottles. You don't have to remember to take anything with you when you go out. You don't have to get out of your seat (or your bed) to get anything when your baby is hungry. You have food available instantly, whenever it's needed.

The very nature of breastfeeding means that it's an obligatory moment of physical closeness. You can't get somebody else to feed your baby while you get on with your chores; you have to stop for a moment and touch. Actually making physical contact with another person is so important, it produces oxytocin and reduces stress.[10] You have to take that moment with your baby when you breastfeed; you have to connect.

Breastfeeding often calms down a cross baby, or a toddler with a tantrum, pretty quickly, so breastfed babies are generally quiet babies. It's a quick solution to most problems, whether that be a hungry baby, or one that is tired, overwhelmed, scared or goodness knows what else.

Formula is expensive. Using it can cost upwards of £350 a year just for the milk, depending on the brand and type.[11] Although you can spend money on breastfeeding (buying accessories) there is no need for anything except a little bit more food for the mother and, perhaps, a couple of breast pads.

There are more global benefits to breastfeeding that extend to our communities and beyond. An often overlooked benefit of breastfeeding is that it begets more breastfeeding. If your mother breastfed you, then you're more likely to plan to breastfeed[12] and if you see breastfeeding around you then you are also more likely to breastfeed.[13] The more people do it, the more we talk about it; the more we show it, the more it happens. Breastfeeding can help to cause a ripple effect, to help other people to have easier breastfeeding journeys themselves.

We live in a world where we're continually told about environmental issues and taught to do our best to avoid them. Breastfeeding has a very low impact environmentally since you need so little to do it. Although you can buy accessories for breastfeeding such as specially designed clothes, breast pumps or breastfeeding covers, you don't *have* to. The only necessary equipment is attached to your body and only needs a few extra calories of food to fuel the process.

Formula, on the other hand, needs to be manufactured. It's derived from cow's milk so there is an environmental cost from farming. It's then packaged which carries its own environmental cost in manufacture and disposal. Transporting the goods around the world also has environmental consequences. We then add plastic bottles with rubber teats, which also need to be made and disposed of, as well as washed. Plastic waste, in particular, is a big environmental concern since it takes so long to break down and recycling can be limited. Many people use some form of steriliser, some of which use electricity. We have accessories such as bottle warmers or automated formula machines. Ultimately, formula use is more detrimental to the environment.

So why bother to breastfeed? It's healthier, more intimate, cheaper, better for the environment, and it sets a helpful example for other new mothers. While it can be hard, when it works it's so worth it.

20

LEARNING TO LOVE BREASTFEEDING

I was adamant I would only breastfeed for six months. I believed in its value, but I didn't enjoy it. It had been painful, it was hard and it was so time-consuming. I could hardly get any time away from Finlay and, much as I love him, everyone needs some time to themselves every now and again. I looked forward to being able to have a break from the perpetual demands and responsibility.

Now, I know that, up until now, I've spent a lot of time complaining. But I believe that not enough people share their struggles honestly. I love Fin, but being a mother was shockingly hard work and breastfeeding was a significant part of that. The weight of responsibility for being continually on call was such a culture shock. Sure, snuggling up is lovely, but when you're looking at your mountains of ironing it can seem frustratingly time-consuming.

The difficulties which set me off to a bad start were

avoidable. A lot of the things I found daunting would have been easier to face had I realised that so many women find the same things hard, and that everything is transient. I think having a realistic view is more helpful, especially when teamed with a support network of women who can reassure you about what is normal and how to cope with things that are tricky.

The rosy picture that was painted to me about how wonderful breastfeeding and motherhood are was unfair. Babies are lovely, but parenting is hard, *really* hard. Knowing that actually helps you to cope. If you think everything is meant to be wonderful then finding that it's not comes as something of a shock. If you know it can be tough, but that it passes, then that's different.

If you know who to ask or where to go to get help instead of thinking that you should innately be able to breastfeed then it makes a big difference. I'd been fed an image of breastfeeding as continual motherly bliss. This unrealistic expectation doesn't help anybody. I thought I was abnormal.

If I told people I wasn't completely delighted with motherhood they looked at me like I was insane. I felt I was allowed to make jokes about how tired I was, but not to say that, sometimes, I felt bored, or down, or isolated. If I admitted that breastfeeding was arduous then I was told to stop. I couldn't let out my frustrations, which for me is an important part of coping.

It wasn't just me, I know that now. I've talked to enough women to know that it's common. I think we need, as a society, to be more honest and supportive. Being a mother is hard and it's OK to struggle. You don't have to love every single second of the experience, you just have to love the baby.

We shouldn't need to do it alone. Humans aren't designed that way. Sometimes, you might need to let off steam with a friend or you might need somebody to hold the baby while you sleep or bring you a meal you haven't had to struggle to make. Sometimes, you might need someone to say that they struggled too so you don't feel alone. We need each other.

When Fin was three months old I was looking for a new book to read. I'd devoured hundreds of novels in the hours spent sitting around with a baby in my arms, usually attached to my breasts. I decided that I wanted to read a bit about breastfeeding. I wasn't looking for a 'how-to' book, because by then I was feeling confident I was doing it right; I wanted something meatier. I browsed the internet and found good reviews for a book called *The Politics of Breastfeeding* by Gabrielle Palmer[1] so I ordered a copy.

As I sat and read whilst feeding Fin in my rocking chair my mouth fell open. I finally realised that my story was nothing new. Lots of women were falling foul of a society where breastfeeding is no longer normal. We're subject to marketing ploys and lack of understanding and support. We're living in a predominantly formula-feeding culture where breastfeeding has fallen to endangered levels. No wonder I'd struggled.

Nothing that had happened had been my fault and I wasn't alone; there were so many struggling women out there. When I realised the history and breadth of issues that injure breastfeeding I felt it was a wonder I'd stuck with it;

my stubbornness can be of benefit sometimes. In fact, I had a lot to be proud of. I'd withstood the social pressures that shook my foundations; the lack of support, the poor advice, the judgement and the constant threat of a bottle. I was breastfeeding in a society that wasn't conducive to it and I'd done it!

Reading that book took me back to that antenatal breastfeeding workshop. On the day I'd first become interested in breastfeeding and become aware that it wasn't as straightforward as I'd thought. This felt like the next awakening; from awareness to comprehension.

I was so angry. Nobody should have to struggle with their biology as a result of politics. If you want to breastfeed then you should be able to. It's disgusting that babies die and women hurt because of this stupid mess we're in. There's a lack of information before birth (I was lucky to have had 'so much', a whole day!), lack of exposure to breastfeeding, lack of support after birth, poor understanding from health professionals, discomfort surrounding breastfeeding in public and a dearth of experience, information and understanding in the community. It's a miracle that anyone manages it. One thing was for sure, I wanted to help, if even in the tiniest way.

It was then that I wrote the preface to this book, one evening after finishing *The Politics of Breastfeeding*. I didn't know where I was going with it but I knew I wanted to write it down. I wanted to tell the story of breastfeeding in a world where it's not commonplace, like waving a little flag and shouting, 'We're here!' I wanted to tell it for what it is, warts and all; not a pretty picture to try and lure people into giving it a go, but a real story of what it's like, why it matters and why we should care.

I distinctly remember when I decided I was going to breastfeed for longer than six months. I was in the car with my friend, Helen, who had a slightly older baby. We were on the way home from a play date with another mutual friend and were chatting about our babies on the way home.

'Well, Fin's five months old now. I'm going to stop at six months,' I said

'Oh? I never got on with breastfeeding myself. We put our daughter on formula in hospital,' Helen said.

'Yeah, I remember you saying. Well, I'm done too now. On his six month birthday I'm locking myself away without a phone. Somebody else will have to get up and feed him day and night. I'm going to sleep,' I joked. This was a fantasy that got me get through some of the rough days. But as I told Helen I began to *really* visualise what it would be like. Not the peace and sleep, that still held some appeal, but *stopping* breastfeeding. A lump formed in my throat, much to my surprise.

Over the next few days I mulled this over. I realised that I didn't want to stop breastfeeding and I had even started to *enjoy* it. This was quite an epiphany. Despite everything I'd been through, maybe even because of it, I was now in love with breastfeeding. It had happened so gradually I hadn't even noticed.

I actually liked that Finlay was wholly dependent on me. I knew him like nobody else. I kind of enjoyed those bleary-eyed moments in the middle of the night when we were totally alone and peace and quiet reigned. I liked the lifestyle breastfeeding had led to of attachment parenting, catering to my baby's needs in an intricate dance that taught me everything about him. Above all, though, I was tremendously proud of myself. I had fought through the difficulties, and here I was, still doing it. What had once been fraught had started to become *easy,* even enjoyable!

I began to value the benefits of breastfeeding so much. For a start, I never had to worry about sterilising or packing bottles. I'm not the most organised person, probably because I am always doing far too many things to hold in my head at once. I can guarantee I would have frequently gone out without enough milk if it wasn't stored in my bra. As it was, I was often begging for nappies, wipes and spare clothes.

When Fin wanted a feed I didn't have to get up and go and sort out a bottle, I could just pop him 'on the boob' without much thought. I'd stopped thinking about whether he was 'due a feed' and would solve every problem by breastfeeding. It was a relaxed way to parent. My mum once said that if breastfeeding had been that laid back when she was doing it then she would have carried on for a lot longer.

I knew that I was everything to Finlay. With everybody else constantly clamouring for a bit of baby attention it gave me something that put me above everyone else. I had birthed him and I sustained him. I was the most important thing in *his* life, even if I felt disregarded by the friends that I once thought held me important too.

I think, with your first child, it can be hard to see your way out of the woods. Eventually, of course, you will get elements of your old identity back. One day I would be able to go out with my friends, go to work or go to rehearsals with my band. It's hard to see that in the never-ending days with a newborn. I felt like everything I had been, everything that defined me, was gone. So, even though I loved Fin intensely, I also felt stuck. I resented everyone else who was able to coo at the baby and then go back to their lives. This included Stuart, who got to leave the house and be one person while I was always two; even in my sleep.

Now, however, I saw that breastfeeding kept me inextricably linked to my baby. Initially, it had made me feel trapped. Before Fin was born I'd done what I wanted, when I wanted. I had this hectic social life filled with hobbies and projects; I went out three nights a week for karate training and at least once a week I would be out singing. Poor Stuart barely saw me once you factored in work and evenings out with friends. I knew when we had a baby things would change, but I don't think I realised the extent. I couldn't have a few minutes to strum a guitar or to do a work-out, let alone go out to a rehearsal or a karate session. Everything I did, I did with Fin. I had a perpetual feeling of having a mind functioning at double time, one half thinking of what I needed or wanted, and half thinking about him. I'd never had to think this way before; I had never spent much time thinking about anybody else's needs.

I'm the kind of person who agrees to things. If somebody suggests I do something I will generally be up for it. My hobbies and social life meant a lot to me and did a lot to keep stoking my ego. I know that, if I had formula-fed, I would have been out. I would have agreed to the nights out and I'd have been back doing karate, telling Stuart that I needed the headspace. I deserved some 'me-time', I'm not suggesting otherwise, but I know myself well. I would have taken it to extremes; I always have done. I would have handed Stuart the baby and been off at times when we should have been sharing the workload. I'm not suggesting, for a moment, that that is what mums who formula feed do. It's just what *I* would have done. Being tied to Fin day and night, although it was hard, made me, for the first time, not prioritise my own desires. It made me a better mother and a better person. It has to be one of the best things that came from breastfeeding; the way that he became like a part of my body; the way that he forced me to be there for him, always. It may have been a hard transition but it was one that I came to value.

As it happened, I had lost most of the weight I had put on, too. Although I had lost some of the muscle tone from regular karate training, I was now fitting back in my old clothes and feeling good about what I saw in the mirror. But more to the point, I now recognised that my body's worth wasn't dependent on its aesthetics. I had grown, birthed and sustained a baby with my own, imperfect body. The little things that I had hang-ups about didn't matter any more. I looked in the mirror and saw something amazing.

I started to take my self-worth from being a good mother, instead of being a show off at a gig or doing well at work. I stopped trying to do everything and focussed on what was important. I could exercise without going to karate, I could sing without it being for an audience (nursery rhymes are singing, too). Perhaps this transition to motherhood was tough on me because it was such a complete change. But, actually, it was one that I needed.

Despite my antipathy towards long-term breastfeeding, I had always found the science fascinating, the way that it nourishes and protects babies is just amazing. Seeing it in action is incredible, watching your baby grow and thrive because of your milk. It helped me to feel like I was doing something when Fin was poorly, too, just feeding him was helping him heal.

When Fin was a newborn his eye went crusty. My perfect baby had a defect. (Well, I say perfect, he also had lots of milia or milk spots, when he was born and did, I suppose, look a bit purple, squashed and gross to other people). As usual, I was thinking the worst and was worried sick he might end up blind. I showed it to my midwife who gave me some reassurance and said it would clear up, being a fairly common occurrence with babies.

Anyway, I did my usual internet search and found people suggesting putting breast milk on it. I'd been using water to clean his eye but the crustiness would always come back. So, rather than soak the cotton wool I'd been using to clean his eye with water I expressed a little milk on to it instead.

Now, I'm not going to say this was a magic cure, it's not like there was a little puff of smoke and the infection vanished. But, within a day, it had almost gone. Of course, this could have been purely coincidental, but I don't think so given breast milk's anti-infective properties.

Breast milk was my new cure-all. It went on burns, cuts, grazes…I'm certain it helped but the main thing it dealt with was my cracked nipples. It did the trick when nothing else was working.

I didn't inflict my new medicine on anybody else. I'm pretty sure most people would have thought it was gross and weird.

'I burnt myself on the oven last night.'

'Ooo, I can help. Hold still while I squirt some milk on that.' No, I think I would lose friends that way.

As time went on, I began to find bottle-feeding rather alien. As a girl it had been a normal part of my experience, everyone I knew used formula and I bottle fed my own sister. But, now that breastfeeding was normal to me, something that I did perhaps ten to fifteen times a day, bottle-feeding seemed weird. I would feel utterly perplexed when hearing mothers anxiously discussing how many ounces their babies had drunk or should have drunk. I had no concept at all of how much Fin had drunk, all I knew was whether he seemed sated and whether he filled his nappy.

I would go so far as to say I was anti-formula for a while. I hate that I'm saying that. I like to think that I 'live and let live'. But, on reflection, although I hope that it isn't something I ever expressed, I felt negative about formula feeding. I felt uneasy when I saw babies being formula-fed. I would feel sad and wonder 'what went wrong'. It took a while of hearing my peers' stories to fully understand that every woman does the best for her baby in her particular circumstances. It wasn't my business to even have an opinion.

On a personal level, I was terrified about the prospect of my baby being given formula behind my back and would be furious at the suggestion that I would ever allow a drop to pass his lips for any reason. There were many times when formula could have made my life 'easier' (such as if it improved sleep or gave me a break), but I had continually fought my corner and won. Giving formula was like giving in to me, and I'm too stubborn for that. I worried that if I was away for a short time others would give my baby formula out of ignorance of just how much breastfeeding meant to me. It went beyond feeding; it was heavily wrapped up with my parenting experience.

I had to protect breastfeeding, as if it was a child in its own right, growling like a mother bear any time anybody threatened this weak infant that I named 'Breastfeeding'. As time went on and Breastfeeding grew healthier I could relax. I began to see that others around me could be hurt by the things I said or did in defence of breastfeeding, and that I needed to open my eyes to their feelings too.

I started to truly see that my formula feeding friends were also super-mums. Some had tried to breastfeed and got into horrid situations that had forced them to stop. Others had never wanted to breastfeed in the first place. Where, at one point, I would fervently wish that my friends would get the support they needed, or feel heartbroken that things hadn't worked out for them, I began to see that this standpoint was unkind. We all have the right to walk our own path and their decision to formula feed didn't endanger my decision to breastfeed. Instead, I could be protective of them also. I could be angry with the social situation that landed us all in this mess, but I should have nothing but support for my fellow mothers. My love for breastfeeding should extend to recognition of the struggle for all mothers.

I think it's common to feel this way with any passionate new love. Similarly, when I first got into karate I thought all other martial arts were a waste of time. Karate was the 'right' one. But I got to a point where I was proficient at it and had become friendly with other martial artists and would share ideas with them. I didn't need to be defensive any more. With formula feeding mums I could listen to their stories and empathise. This wouldn't make me switch to formula any more than hanging out with a Sikh would make me convert from Christianity; I was secure now.

I know that mums, in that defensive phase, can wound one another; is it any wonder when we're placed under so much pressure? I'm sure it was something I did unintentionally and that I was certainly on the receiving end of a few times. Looking back, I can see that the in-fighting with mums is simply because they are so passionate about what they do. It's a demonstration of deep love and protection for their vulnerable, hard-won situations. I don't know whether it's a phase that has to occur in order to come out of the other side, I'm no psychologist. But I've made peace with my own feelings. Whilst I may care about better support and awareness of breastfeeding that doesn't mean that I want formula feeders to be marginalised or that I feel sorry for them. Every mum deserves support and empowerment.

While I came to terms with my new passion for breastfeeding I thought more about my own breastfeeding journey. I decided that my plan would be to have no plan. I would try to breastfeed for two years or more, but essentially I would just do it until I stopped.

One day I was at Helen's house. She was describing somebody she thought I might know.

'You know, she's one of those nutters who breastfeed for a really long time,' she said. I didn't react. I saw the thought processes show in her face when she realised she had no idea of my intentions or my opinions on extended breastfeeding.

'You won't be one of those, will you?' she asked, looking panicked.

'Who knows, probably,' I answered smiling. It had stopped mattering what other people thought of my parenting decisions. I knew I was doing OK, taking it all day by day. This was such a change in opinion from how I had felt early on when I was counting down the days. For me now, breastfeeding was a normal part of life.

Seemingly to keep me on my toes, a new breastfeeding problem developed. Fin started to bite. I read about it and found some people on forums suggesting that if you yelp it would scare them and stop them from doing it. But no, Fin thought my crying out with pain was hilarious and he'd do it again. I was at a loss because I didn't want to have new problems after things had just started to get good.

I thought about what I had learned from my experiences; I knew exactly what to do. For the first time in my breastfeeding experience I would actually ask for help.

I'd held off from going to my local breastfeeding support group because I think I'd failed to understand the word 'support'. Although the group had been highly recommended by my midwife I'd assumed it was a sort of breastfeeding club, one that you joined when you were a seasoned hippy, not a fraud like I felt I was.

I first went to the group when Fin was three months old and discovered that it wasn't at all what I expected. They were a warm group of mums who I could talk to about the trials and tribulations of breastfeeding and actually be understood. I wasn't the alien any more, these mums felt the same pressures and had helpful tips to get you through the day. Ruth, the midwife from my antenatal class, ran the group and was on hand anytime anyone had a pressing question. It was time to get help.

I was nervous going to group that day, I felt like I was going to be sick. Even though I'd attended the group regularly, today was different. When Ruth came by and chatted to me, I plucked up my courage.

'Ruth, I wanted to ask you something,' I said. My cheeks flushed. 'Finlay keeps biting me and I don't know what to do. I tried yelping but he thinks it's funny…' I trailed off. Ruth smiled gently.

'Well, the thing to do is to look for a cue that tells you he's going to bite and take him away before it happens, to break the cycle. Unfortunately, your crying out is encouraging him. If he does do it, take him away from the breast for thirty seconds. He'll soon learn the connection that biting means no milk.'

'Thanks, I'll give it a go,' I said with relief.

Of course, motherhood being what it is, Fin didn't do it again that night. But the very next time that he did, I followed Ruth's suggestion and it worked perfectly. I was so glad I had asked, getting an easy solution to the problem instead of potentially months of battling. I felt a pang that I hadn't done this many times before.

I was in a good place now. I felt confident about my

ability to breastfeed and I was passionate about its importance. I had found an understanding and encouraging community at my local support group who helped me to feel normal. I could talk about how I felt without fear of judgement; I allowed myself to admit that I found some things hard. I allowed myself to ask for help because I knew that I was asking people who understood how I was feeling.

I was *happy*. I was proud of the choices I had made and fought for. I was enjoying my parenting journey and getting so much fulfilment from trying to be a supportive friend to other mothers treading a similar road to the one I'd travelled.

Breastfeeding didn't need an end date. It was as routine a part of my day as checking my social media updates. One day, it would come to an end and that would be a sad signal that my son was growing up. Until then, I would continue to grow him with my body, just as I had whilst pregnant. I was his for as long as he wanted me.

21

WEANING

All good things must come to an end. Humans can't live on breast milk forever; eventually we must be weaned.

When you wean somebody off something, you reduce their reliance on it. The word comes from the Anglo-Saxon 'wenian' which means 'to become accustomed to something else'.[1] Weaning from breast milk starts when solids are introduced, when a baby starts to get nutrients from other sources in addition to breast milk. Over time, the baby shifts their needs more on to solid food until, eventually, they stop breastfeeding altogether.

As I've already said, the recommended age to start giving a baby solid food is six months. At this point the baby should be showing signs that they're ready for 'real' food: they should be able to sit up; to grasp food, put it in their mouth and swallow it.[2(p22)] Before babies are ready to be weaned they have a tongue-thrust reflex where they push anything put into their mouth out with their tongue. After four months this reflex begins to disappear.[2(p57)] So, when a baby can steal your food and eat it, they're ready to be weaned. Altogether it makes sense that when a baby is ready developmentally they ought to be ready physically. It would be a pretty bad design otherwise.

As with anything else, I find it useful to think in terms of what humans would do without all the trappings of society. I suppose a baby would start to take food from their parents when they were ready. Perhaps they would be given bits of food to feel and play with. Our ancestors wouldn't be strapping babies into a chair and shovelling in liquidised food.

Back when I had been weaned, in 1984, the advice was to start giving solids at four months.[3] It's now thought that babies' digestive systems aren't ready that early. Starting solids later reduces the risk of allergies and illness because before six months babies may still have an 'open gut'.[4,5] The cells of their guts are spaced out so that larger molecules like antibodies can pass into the blood, but it means that macromolecules from foods can also do so and the body may not be ready for that.

Traditional baby foods would have included baby rice and rusks,[2(p28)] neither of which is particularly nutritionally beneficial to a baby.[6] Baby rice is finely milled rice that can be mixed with milk to make a gloopy, easily spooned, foodstuff and rusks are basically very crumbly biscuits. Aside from that, babies were given pureed food since they were too young to chew. Then, as they got older, their food would contain more lumps.[5]

Introducing solid food early means that a baby has less room in their tummy for breast milk. Breast milk is more calorific than solid foods so this has an impact on infant weight gain.[7(p37)] It also has a better balance of nutrients.[6]

Early weaning can lead to more infections due to exposure to unhygienic feeding utensils and reduction in antibodies from breast milk.[7(pp30-31)] Quite simply, it's too young.

As with anything related to parenting it seems, introducing solids has become politicised. Historically babies were weaned later, usually much older than six months.[8] The first commercial baby food, 'Clapp's baby soup', was made in 1921.[7(p22)] It was essentially a beef broth and had some moderate success. This paved the way for the still ubiquitous Gerber baby foods (now owned by Nestlé), supposedly created in 1928 by Daniel Gerber because his wife was exhausted from hand-straining vegetables for the baby.[7(p22)] Gerber foods were marketed as convenient and more nutritious than home-made foods; these selling points led to it becoming extremely popular in a matter of a few years.[7(p23)]

Of course, introducing complementary foods earlier has an economic benefit to the companies that make them commercially. Complementary foods were being marketed heavily and mothers began to believe they were needed from a young age.[7(p23)] By the 1970s, babies only a few weeks old were being fed baby foods; the majority by three months.[9] A three month baby is developmentally so young. They are only just leaving the 'fourth trimester', the phase where babies transition from womb to world. Where a six-month-old baby can sit up and grab at things they want, a three-month-old spends most of their time laying down and can do little more than smile.

The nutritional claims and labelling of baby foods started to come under fire and, together with research conducted in the meantime, led to the recommendation in 2001 that solids should not be introduced until six months.[10] Although this is a highly controversial area of science (with many papers being financially backed by baby food manufacturers)[7(p31)] the upshot is that there is no harm in waiting to wean and it does appear to reduce the risk of gastrointestinal infections.[11] In the meantime, breast milk or formula milk provide a balance of nutrients and plenty of calories.

The approach to introducing solids was beginning to change when I had Fin. Gill Rapley and Tracey Murkett had not long released their book *Baby-led Weaning*[2] and the idea was quickly taking hold. In baby-led weaning, instead of spooning pureed food into a baby's mouth, you offer a variety of foods for the baby to feed themselves. So, you might give soft fruits, cooked vegetables, fingers of toast or anything easy to grasp and safe to gum on. Babies can explore the foods themselves, making decisions about what to try and when. Some people worry about the baby choking on these kinds of foods, but actually babies have a strong gagging reflex and it helps them to learn about which foods can be swallowed (anything posing a real choking hazard, like nuts or whole grapes shouldn't be given to a baby).[2(pp61-63)]

The process is messy but, ultimately, it allows babies to set the pace, which makes complete sense to me. As with so many things with parenting it's a case of knowing your baby and following your and their instincts. Somebody once explained it to me that, as an adult, you wouldn't want somebody spooning runny food into your mouth with you having little means to communicate with them when you need more time to swallow or when you need to slow down. Surely, it must be similar for a baby; feeding themselves must be a more pleasurable and interesting experience.

At six months a baby only needs 196 calories a day from solids, increasing to 455 by the time they are nine to twelve months old.[12] This isn't a lot and offering a baby a variety of solids can meet this need. After around six months babies' nutrient stores start to deplete, so a range of complementary foods becomes important.[2(p35)]

Only two nutrients complicate that matter. Here in the Northern Hemisphere, vitamin D is in short supply. We make vitamin D through our skin being exposed to sunlight, just thirty minutes a day making enough.[2(p40)] In the British winter we only see the sun for eight hours a day and spend most of that time indoors or huddled in winter clothing. Most people don't get enough vitamin D under these conditions. For that reason, it's advisable for pregnant and breastfeeding mothers to take vitamin D supplements.[2(p40)]

Iron can also be a complicated matter. Breast milk is sometimes reported as being deficient in iron because it contains lower quantities than formula, however, iron (as with other nutrients) is more bioavailable in breast milk.[13] Less is needed since the baby can absorb it more readily. This said, the baby's stores of iron do get lower as they get older and, after six months, iron is needed from other sources. Therefore, iron rich complementary foods are advisable in the early days.[2(pp144-145)]

Regardless, breast milk continues to contribute an important part of the diet until the baby is fully dependent on solid foods at two years or older. Formula-fed babies can be moved on to cow's milk at a year if they are eating well.[14]

The word 'weaning' can also be applied to when breastfeeding comes to an end. Naturally, this would be a gradual process, with the baby demanding more as their reliance on solids increases. I suppose weaning is a journey, perhaps starting when solids are introduced. Maybe the journey starts sooner, when the total dependence of a newborn on its mother begins to shift, such as when a mother expresses milk for another caregiver to feed the baby. Whatever the semantics, a baby's reduced reliance on breastfeeding can be bittersweet.

22

TAKING THE BACK SEAT

As much as I was protective over breastfeeding, I did have to start to relinquish control. The first steps towards this began when Fin was three months old.

I was, I confess, jealous at times of my bottle-feeding friends who reported being able to leave their baby at a few months old. I, on the other hand, was firmly tied to my offspring. I could only escape for such small periods of time that it wasn't worth bothering. Fin felt like a part of me, like an arm or a leg.

I have an involved husband and an enthusiastic family who wanted to help out so it wasn't that I didn't have the support, or necessarily that I didn't want it. But Fin needed milk and I was the source of that.

I knew, eventually, I would have to leave Fin. I craved simple things like going to the cinema. It seems silly, but it can be so frustrating when you can no longer do small, normal things. I wasn't going to risk having an upset baby for the sake of a film but I wanted some escapism, some sense of my pre-mum self. I wanted to be able to go out, on occasion, and I would, eventually, need to go back to work (although that was a long way off). My little limpet would need to find other rocks to cling to once in a while.

When Fin was four months old freedom was forced upon me. I was going to be returning to university in the evenings to study a part-time Master's degree that I'd started before I became pregnant. I had taken a term's break while Fin was tiny naively thinking that, after that, he would be old enough for me to go out once a week.

How wrong I was. The idea of Fin getting milk without me and going to sleep without me feeding him to sleep seemed impossible. We had a month from when my place was confirmed on my course to ease him into it. It was time to begin work.

Before Fin was born I'd bought some of the accoutrements of bottle-feeding 'just in case', or for when I wanted to express milk. I had some bottles that, according to the label, were designed to be compatible with breastfeeding and I had a steriliser. I didn't buy a breast pump because I figured I would express milk by hand. I also didn't buy any formula; it had seemed enough like tempting fate to be buying bottles without also having formula in the house. In this day and age of continual shop opening, I wasn't going to be without formula milk if it transpired I needed it. Looking back, if we'd had a tin of formula in the house I'm fairly certain Stuart would have fought to use it so, for us, it was a good decision not to buy any. I never even used my steriliser, in fact it stayed in a dusty box under the stairs until we sold it.

I was resolute not to give Fin a bottle until, or unless, I absolutely had to. I wanted to avoid nipple confusion and I also didn't want to faff about with expressing milk needlessly. I know family members would have loved to feed him and, had they have seen a bottle in use, would have jumped at the chance. But I think we need to get out of the mindset that feeding a baby is something that people do as part of their bonding experience. If the baby is breastfed someone else feeding them is off the table.

Anyway, the first step towards leaving Fin was to get to grips with expressing milk by hand. It looked easy enough from the pictures and I wasn't fussed about it being time-consuming. I wanted to build up a stash of milk in the freezer (where it keeps for six months) so there was no worry about running out.

One evening, when Stuart was out, I decided to give it a try. Expressing in front of Stuart made me feel really uncomfortable; it seemed compromising, squirting milk out like a dairy cow. I sterilised a bowl to use (milk sprays out of your nipple like water from a shower-head so I found it easier to catch it in a large receptacle) and thoroughly washed my hands. I stuck something mundane on the TV and settled down to have a go.

The milk began to flow fairly quickly. I had to keep swapping sides as the milk would slow and my hands start to ache. Every few minutes, I tipped the milk I had produced into a little breast milk bag. These bags come sterilised and have measuring lines up the side so you can see how much you've put in. I would feel like I had produced loads of milk but then, when it was poured into the bag, it would only be a few millilitres. It was slow going and I produced a meagre offering.

The trouble with expressing milk is that your body is so attuned to the needs of your baby that there isn't a lot extra to express. Also, a baby is far better at getting the milk out than your hand or a breast pump.[1] I realised I was going to have to express milk quite a few times to have a satisfactory amount stored. I was proud, nonetheless, and put the bag in the freezer, carefully labelled.

The next time I expressed I kept the milk and didn't freeze it. Stuart and I sterilised one of Fin's bottles with boiling water and then poured in the milk. It was emotional for both of us, I think. For me, it was hard to relinquish the one thing that nobody else could do for Fin. For Stuart, it was momentous to be providing sustenance for his son.

I hovered around to help if needed, trying to stay out of sight in case it was a problem if Fin saw me. I was anxious as the false teat went into my baby's mouth. But Fin was having none of it; he hardly even sucked. He screeched with clenched fists whenever the bottle touched his lips. In a way I was thrilled that Fin hadn't suddenly loved the bottle and dismissed my services. On the other, how on earth was I ever going to get away from him? Would I have to quit my degree? Would I have to quit work? Should I shackle myself to this little dictator for perpetuity?

We tried everything we could think of. Stuart fed Fin, I fed him, my mother fed him…I was tempted to let the binman in for a go. We tried warm milk, cold milk, and hot milk. We tried holding Fin tummy-to-tummy like he was being breastfed, or lying on his back, or sitting up, or even not holding him at all and sitting him in a bouncy chair. I tried breastfeeding Fin and then launching a sneak attack with the bottle. It was all to no avail and a lot of hard expressed milk went down the sink.

Expressing regularly by hand was time-consuming, so, I bought a manual breast pump. It had a conical flange that fitted over my breast. When I pressed a handle it created a suction that drew my nipple into a tunnel, which would make some milk squirt out. This milk would drip into a bottle, which could be unscrewed and attached to a teat or emptied into a bag, whichever I preferred. It was quicker and easier than hand expressing so I used it every time I needed to express milk.

I wanted to see if things would be different if I wasn't there and to give Stuart the opportunity to experiment without my continual supervision. We agreed a date when I would leave him in charge.

I fretted about the details. The milk was ready and stored up. Stuart had been suitably nagged with every bit of advice I could think of. I wallowed in guilt because I knew this was all to prepare for me to leave Fin for non-essential reasons; I could have deferred my degree for longer and then the pressure would have been off. I'd been clueless as to how dependent a breastfed baby is on their mother. I'd thought somebody could give him a bottle; other babies seem to be OK with it. The idea of a baby not wanting a bottle was a new one on me.

The day inevitably came. I dragged myself reluctantly out of the house to go for a walk, staying in the area in case Stuart needed me. It was a glorious summer's day so I strolled towards the beach. As I neared the sea I began to feel a draw to my old friend. This time I wasn't trudging there with a baby strapped to my front, determined to lose weight, I was 'taking a break', letting somebody else shoulder my burden. I broke into a run. I was responsibility-free; just one brain inside my head. I sank down on to a rock by the shore with a lump in my throat. I sat and drank in the freedom, having learnt what it means to be perpetually responsible.

Soon the agreed time was up. I had left Fin for almost two hours, far longer than ever before. As I started walking uphill to my house thoughts of Fin flooded back. It didn't weigh me back down; it was my chores that did that, not my incredible son. I was excited to see him. My pace quickened the closer I got as anxious thoughts swirled in my mind. Had Fin cried? Was he hungry? Would Stuart have coped?

I burst through the door of my house and ran to find Fin. Stuart looked decidedly frazzled but Fin looked perfectly happy. He hadn't wanted his bottle, no matter what Stuart tried, but he'd managed to distract him with games. At least I now knew the world didn't end if I popped out but we still had to solve the issue of feeding.

Again, at the end of my tether, (having haemorrhaged money on every type of bottle teat I could think of) I put a plea on Facebook for ideas. I felt sure *somebody* must have had a similarly boob-obsessed baby.

A few friends came back with the idea of using a cup. I knew that cups (as opposed to bottles) could be used to reduce the risk of nipple confusion in newborns.[2] Nonetheless, it hadn't occurred to me to try it with an older child. I looked into the matter and came across the *Doidy cup*. These are open-topped and have slanted sides. The baby can lap or sip the milk up as you tilt the cup, but due to the slant you can both see the milk coming, meaning that you can more easily control how much you tip towards the baby. Since toddlers can use them I figured I would use it eventually, one way or another, so it wouldn't be a total waste of money. I bought one in bright yellow (my favourite colour) and eagerly awaited its arrival.

When the cup came in the post I immediately sterilised it with boiling water and poured some milk in. I sat Finlay up and gently tipped the milk into his mouth. He enthusiastically lapped it up. Sometimes, he got too big a gulp and coughed, but that was my fault, I had to learn how to get the tilt just right. Fin got a lot down his front but still, he was feeding *happily* from a source other than my breasts. I was understandably elated.

Stuart didn't like it. He found cup-feeding messy and awkward. He was convinced that Fin was hardly getting any milk inside him. I tried to persuade Stuart to persevere but he just didn't get on with it. Of course, he had every right to his own opinions, but I was getting very anxious about my impending need to leave Fin. So much hinged on the success of this little cup! It was irrelevant that I liked it as a method because I could breastfeed Fin. Stuart decided to keep trying bottles.

We still needed to tackle the other obstacle to my going out, which was that of sleep. Leaving Fin when he was awake and happy was an entirely different issue to leaving him in the evening (which I was going to be doing), when he would be tired and crabby. Sleep was inextricably linked to breastfeeding. When Fin was tired he would only be comforted by breastfeeding and he would scream the house down if we tried to fob him off with anything else

I experimented with getting Fin to sleep in other ways. As long as he had a full belly he could be rocked to sleep in my arms. Sometimes, if he had a dummy, he would drift off in his cot if I sat holding his hands.

I passed on my experiences to Stuart who willingly gave it a try, making me promise that I wouldn't interfere. I sat downstairs and listened to the familiar routine of bath time, getting pyjamas on and a story. Then I listened to Fin crying inconsolably while his dad tried to get him to sleep without milk, anxiously watching the minutes tick by on the clock. I decided I couldn't take any more. I had made the decision long ago that Fin wasn't going to cry himself to sleep; I couldn't let it happen now.

I started creeping up the stairs and the crying quietened. I hesitated; it had gone quiet. I sat on the stairs and waited, straining to hear any sound. After a while, Stuart appeared, looking guilty. He'd got Fin to sleep, but he'd been sobbing quietly the whole time. This broke my heart even though he'd been in his loving father's arms, which is an entirely different scenario to a baby left alone. Still, I couldn't wait for him to wake for his next feed so that I could cuddle him to apologise for allowing this trauma. It seemed that, whereas I could ease Fin to sleep, Stuart didn't have the knack yet.

So, with a baby that hated bottles and couldn't get to sleep happily without me I went to a lecture, feeling like the worst mum in the world. In retrospect, I'm sure I could have deferred but, at the time, I felt like things would never change and Fin would always need me there. I suppose I thought Stuart would work it out without me there. He wasn't the first dad to be left holding the baby.

In the end, I tried not to think about it. After giving Fin as long a feed as I could, before I left, I beseeched Stuart to call me if Fin was upset so I could come home and help; Stuart wasn't to let him cry himself to sleep. If Stuart had to take him for a drive, or rock him, or get him up and wait for me to get home that was fine.

Stuart tried everything over those eight weeks of once a week lectures. I would come home to either the sound of continued cries, or to a stressed out husband and a little boy sobbing in his sleep and I would fly up the stairs to beg Fin's forgiveness. It was awful but I felt there wasn't an alternative. I had wrongly assumed that we would have this figured out and I'd paid a lot of money for the course.

Fortunately, the lectures were few and I went back to ensuring I was always there at bedtime. But I knew next term we would be back in the same situation, although this time we would have an older baby.

As it transpired, this made a world of difference. When I returned to my course with a seven-month-old baby I would invariably come home to find Fin asleep slumped against his dad. Stuart had discovered that Fin would 'zone-out' if he put cartoons on and would have a little bit of milk from his bottle and then doze off, something he nicknamed a 'pyjama party'. It wasn't ideal, but it wasn't often and it was a lot better than Fin crying himself to sleep.

Next came a big step, I was going to leave him at night with somebody other than his dad; his gran, Angela. This took a lot of trust from me because whereas Stuart had been a part of the saga at bedtime, Fin's gran hadn't. Also, Angela was my mother-in-law, not my mother, and that makes it a bigger leap of faith. I know she loves Fin unequivocally, but I also knew that she and I are different. I knew his well-being would be paramount to her so I tried to not be completely uptight, but I still worried that she would go against my wishes, in some way, or that she would rather struggle with him by herself than call one of us back if Fin was inconsolable. However, it needed to be done. I had to go to a lecture, Stuart had to work a night shift, and I had to trust somebody.

I went out feeling the usual anxiety and apprehension, having reeled off a list of instructions before I left. When, after my lecture, I texted to say I was on my way home, I got a reply to say that he was up having a pyjama party. This use of our little family term made me smile.

I walked in the door to find Fin wide-eyed and full of beans. He had happily drunk his milk from a bottle, having now decided that he didn't mind them but, instead of going to bed, had preferred to lie on the sofa kicking Angela and giggling. I carried Fin upstairs for a quiet breastfeed and he was asleep in minutes.

I could relax knowing that Fin could be left with family. I was free, if I wanted to be. The knowledge I could go out was anathema. I was no longer a prisoner to this most beloved captor.

23

REAL FOOD

I suffered from a milk allergy until I was around eight years old. As a baby I was unsettled and didn't gain weight. Zack claims I cried all the time and my mum says I could 'poo through the eye of a needle'. Once I was on a dairy-free formula (allergies and breastfeeding were poorly understood then) I was better, but solids brought a whole new host of problems for me.

Having a milk problem is harder than you might think. Not being able to have milk wasn't a big deal; I could have soya milk instead. But I also couldn't have butter, cheese, or anything containing dairy products. So many foods contain dairy that it's surprisingly hard to eliminate, especially if you eat food that isn't prepared at home. I remember, even as a small child, reading the backs of packets to make sure they were 'safe'.

It marked me out as different. For instance, I can remember growing cress at school. Everybody else got to try their own cress in egg sandwiches. I had to eat my cress on its own because I was allergic to butter. I'm not sure why

I couldn't have had mine with dry bread, but anyway, pinches of cress weren't too exciting.

Some people were sceptical about my allergy. At the time, it was becoming weirdly trendy to have allergies. I think a lot of people felt Mum was jumping on the bandwagon or being overprotective. It was also before there was widespread understanding of allergies and their implications. Consequently, lots of people used to get me to eat 'forbidden foods', resulting in a lot of time spent vomiting and feeling dreadful.

I did grow out of it, fortunately. At around seven years old I started to try little bits of dairy. I gradually increased my consumption until I discovered I was completely free of my allergy. I'm still a bit allergy prone though; I have hayfever and my skin reacts randomly to all sorts of cosmetics.

Given my history of allergies, and with Stuart also having some sensitivity to dairy, I wanted to do what I could to avoid Fin having similar problems. When I saw that waiting until six months to wean reduced the risk of allergies I was keen to follow the guidance.

Since our parents' generation would have weaned at around four months, understandably, they thought we were waiting too long. They kept telling me how hungry Fin looked and how he would be more settled and sleep better if he started solids. Stuart came home from work with tales of how his colleagues had weaned their children before six months 'and they had turned out alright'. Don't you love that argument? We are told something is bad for us and others retaliate by citing tales of how 'it didn't do them any harm,' seemingly with no concept of the meaning of 'risk'.

My mum friends were suffering the same pressure and some waited while some didn't. Helen felt she'd weaned too early (at four months) and decided to stop solids and start the process again. She told me to follow my instincts. It was reassuring to speak to somebody who felt that they should have waited when I was surrounded by people who said that weaning would be some kind of miracle cure for everything that was difficult with a young baby. Helen was often a source of wise words such as 'it's all a phase' and 'trust your instincts.' She's a far less neurotic mum than I.

So many people suggested that solids would help Fin to sleep. The solution for disrupted sleep had gone from a bottle of formula before bed, to 'cry it out', to food. Each solution suggested there was something wrong with Fin or with the way I was feeding and caring for him, rather than that he was a normal breastfed baby and we had to find ways to cope with that. Again the quality of my milk was being questioned, now it 'wasn't enough for him' and 'if he had some food he would sleep through the night'. Lack of sleep makes your resistance low. It was hard to stick to my guns. Nonetheless, I still fantasised that solids would mean Fin miraculously slept through the night.

When Fin was four months old, I was at the end of my tether. I was up with him five times a night with little respite in the day as he hit the four month sleep regression.[1] I asked my health visitor if this was a sign that I should wean. She quickly reassured me that he was too young and it was a normal developmental stage. It had nothing to do with food. I resolved to remain strong.

Even with ammunition from a health visitor I was still inundated with 'suggestions', to give him a bit of baby rice or some hungry baby milk. It was infuriating! When health visitors were in favour of my baby crying alone in his own room they were to be supported, but when they suggested that I should wait to wean they were to be ignored? Everyone seemed to know best and I was caught in the crossfire.

I was happy to keep up with frequent breastfeeding if I knew it was the right thing to do, but it was hard when people kept making me doubt myself. I had to keep reminding myself that Fin was probably having a growth spurt or, maybe, he just needed to check in with me more often, to be comforted. It didn't have to be about food. Anyway, I would rather prolong the nice (well, if you can use the word 'nice') breastfed baby poo, which smells a bit musty and looks like mustard, and avoid the real stuff for as long as possible!

When Fin was five and a half months old I began to feel, instinctively, that he was ready to have solid food. He fixed me with a steely glare when I ate and would throw himself flailing at my food desperately trying to steal it. I figured the six month guide-line must have some flexibility, since all babies are different, but then I worried I was bending the rules to suit myself.

I decided to consult my health visitor again, this time with Stuart in tow. We undressed Fin and placed him on the white, plastic scales. When his weight was recorded I could see on the chart that it had started to plateau.

'Should I be worried?' I asked.

'No,' she replied, studying the chart. 'It's most likely

because he's into things so much more. At this age they're rolling and grabbing things; they're really active.'

'Is it because he needs solids?' I asked, trying to hide the worry on my face.

'Not necessarily. He's not six months yet is he?'

'Not quite, but he's fascinated by food! I know it might be because he's interested in what I'm doing...' I trailed off.

'Well, you could try the banana test.' Stuart and I glanced at each other to see if either of us showed a flicker of recognition. Seeing our confusion the health visitor carried on. 'You give the baby a piece of banana, they're easy for a baby to hold and nice and soft for their mouth. If he manages to get it in his mouth and swallow it then he's ready to be weaned.'

It seemed so simple, so logical, and I was excited to have got the green light to try.

When we got home I cut up some banana and laid it on Fin's high chair tray. He easily picked up one of the pieces. Stuart and I waited, holding our breaths. Fin put the banana in his eye, his ear and in his hair. He also hit the bulls-eye a few times, seeming to enjoy the taste and little morsels disappeared that must have been swallowed.

That was proof enough for me. I had followed my instincts and waited as long as I felt able given the mounting pressure around me. What more could I do?

I had already bought some baby rice. Although it's fairly nutrient poor, and there's no real reason to start with this, I thought it was 'what you did' since, traditionally, it was the first food for a lot of babies. Although I liked the sound of baby-led weaning I had endured nearly six months of being told that my baby would 'be better once he was on solids'. I had lived through sleepless nights, blending into milk-filled days, and had convinced myself that my baby was hungry; that indeed my milk was not enough. I wanted to ensure that Fin's belly was stuffed to bursting with 'real food', not that he had just had a few licks of a piece of carrot.

I mixed some baby rice with some expressed breast milk as the instructions on the packet said. I started spooning the mixture into Fin's mouth, holding my breath in anticipation. He smacked his lips, churned the food around his mouth and then swallowed. I kept making more and he kept eating it! I began to look forward to my first full night's sleep. Of course, food made absolutely no difference to Fin's sleep, much to the chagrin of my friends and relations...and me.

It goes to show how pointless the anxiety about my milk had been. I wish I had had confidence that I was feeding Fin well with breast milk. I had been full of doubt about my ability to sustain him with my body but he hadn't been hungry; he just wasn't developmentally ready to sleep.

I was excited about Fin's reactions to new tastes and textures so I started to add in new foods. Although I wanted to go slowly so that I could identify if he had a bad reaction to anything, I also wanted to get enough of a variety that he could have three different meals a day as soon as possible. Parsnips were a failure. Yoghurt was a major success. Avocados were tolerated. Each food I tried as a solid for him to hold and mashed up on a spoon for me, experimenting to see what worked for us.

I liked the routine of mealtimes. There had been a time when I ate every meal one handed while I breastfed Fin (he was always hungry at our mealtimes, infuriatingly). Now, he sat in a high chair and Stuart could help if he was at home. It was our first glimpse of a 'family meal time'. It relieved the monotony of mum-life. By the time breakfast was finished, the clearing up was done and a morning nap had been had, it would be lunchtime. Being tired was less of a drag with more to occupy me.

Once we were on to three meals a day (which took a month or so) Fin started to breastfeed less, often only once between meals. I was surprised that he no longer asked for feeds. It was a nice change; it gave me a break and helped to structure the day. Things were more predictable and that afforded me greater freedom.

Fin seemed more content. I felt some people around me wanted to shout 'I told you so!' as if it was proof of my paltry milk. The thing is that breast milk is digested quickly,[2] and so, with solids, it was longer before he wanted something more. My milk had been fine nutritionally. It just didn't keep him full for as long, but that was how it was meant to work. Nothing was wrong.

I was enjoying the changes in life when, at around seven months, I was disgruntled to find my periods were back. Breastfeeding had kept them at bay this long but I suppose that feeding less had changed my hormonal balance and returned my fertility. I felt cheated. I thought about trying to reverse this change by increasing the number of breastfeeds again but this fell by the wayside as I didn't want to offer if Fin didn't ask (although to be fair, he didn't ever refuse). It was a nasty surprise though, after seventeen months of absence.

I wasn't the only one to experience biological changes due to weaning. Finlay had his first real poo. Up until now, he had had typical breastfed baby poo, which, since it's a fairly liquid consistency, tends to be a bit explosive. Visitors cuddling Fin and noticing him looking thoughtful would say in a cutesy voice, 'Oh, I think he's filling his nappy.'

'He isn't,' I would reply.

If they said, 'I think your baby just exploded,' *then* I would fetch the change bag.

Once Fin was weaned he had ordinary, grown-up poo, but the transition seemed difficult. All his first attempts were rock solid and he struggled to get them out. I tried to help by bicycling his legs and massaging his tummy but to no avail. One day, I had left him in the living room and gone upstairs to the toilet. I knew he would stay where I left him because he still wasn't in the least mobile, although I fully expected him to whinge until I came back. My moment of peace was interrupted by a sharp, wounded cry. I panicked, thinking he had somehow pulled something on top of him, and ran down the stairs as fast as I could, to find my little boy red in the face and straining, crying from the pain of his constipation.

I cut down on bananas, toast and other binding foods and gave Fin long breastfeeds to hydrate him. Gradually, it sorted itself out. Now, when visitors tried to accuse Fin of doing a poo we would tell them that, unless he looked like he was giving birth, he wasn't.

I had a new source of paranoia, worrying about what Fin

could, and couldn't, eat. When could he have dairy? Or meat? Or wheat? Or berries? I probably read too much on the subject because it seemed that every food had rules about when it should be introduced. The advice was all so conflicting and there was the ever-present spectre of allergies.

I went for a routine health visitor check when Fin was seven months old.

'How's weaning?' she asked.

'Great! He loves his food! But I'm worried about when he can have certain foods. Should I wait before I give him berries? When can he have dairy? I feel like he'd love to try cheese.'

'Don't worry, other than peanuts and honey, you can give him whatever you want,' she answered. Of course, the guidelines may have changed since then. Still, I felt so relieved that I didn't need to worry. There is so much conflicting information out there, it does get overwhelming.

From then on Fin ate what we ate. I started to give him cow's milk in his porridge, on his cereal or in his food, rather than expressing breast milk for culinary purposes. Whilst I didn't begrudge doing it, if necessary, I was happy to dispense with it once I found that a little cow's milk wouldn't kill him or make him allergic.

Although I felt more confident about what I was feeding him, Fin was a skinny boy. I had always assumed that he took after his tall, slim Dad. But, as I compared him to my friends' babies, I saw that, by far, Fin was the skinniest. This worried me so I went on a mission to fatten Fin up. I desperately wanted to be told at the next health visitor weigh-in that he was bulking up. I also still had in the back of my mind that it might help him to sleep. I shovelled in as much food as I possibly could; three meals a day and snacks in between, as well as breastfeeds on demand.

When I went to see the health visitor she would weigh Fin and record his weight. As time went on the gradient of Fin's measurements was slowly falling off the expected line on the charts. I was quizzed on how much I was feeding him and how good my milk supply was. Of course, I couldn't answer the health visitor's questions; I was just feeding Fin whenever he asked. Without expressing every feed (which wasn't going to happen and is unreliable anyway) I had no way of quantifying what he got. I worried that perhaps my milk was just skimmed.

During these interactions I was never given useful suggestions to improve or assess Fin's intake. I never had a conversation about how often he fed or how many wet and dirty nappies he had. Perhaps I did have issues with producing or transferring enough milk. Perhaps it was the way Fin was meant to be; I will never know. But to this day he remains a long, lean boy.

When Fin was ten months old, Stuart came to Fin's weigh-in. Again, despite me feeding him as much food and milk as I humanly could, he still hadn't gained 'enough'.

'Do you feed your child regular meals?' asked the health visitor

No, I starve him, I thought to myself whilst politely responding, 'Yes, three meals a day and snacks.'

'How much milk does he have?'

'Not a clue,' I glibly replied.

Looking disapprovingly at me, she asked, 'Why not?'

'I breastfeed him,' I answered.

'Oh...right, um...err, well done.' Her cheeks flushed as she fiddled with her paperwork. I could see the panic in her eyes that she couldn't quantify us, she couldn't find out exactly what he was eating. Then, she looked Stuart up and down. 'Well, he's probably slim like your husband. I expect he has a high metabolism,' she said. So what was I then?

Offended, I continued to discuss Fin's development with her. Since he was alert and active she was satisfied, and there was no real discussion about his diet. I remained frustrated that all I ever seemed to do was shovel food into his mouth and yet, inexplicably, he didn't follow the charts.

Of course, weight gain is an important measurement, and I will never know whether Fin was actually being underfed, or if that's just the way he was. But it cannot be that if a breastfed baby doesn't follow the trend it's dismissed as being too difficult to deal with. Even if I concede that Fin should have been heavier; there were never any useful discussions about *breastfeeding*. Since they couldn't check how many ounces of milk Fin was having, it was as if there was nothing that could be done with us so it wasn't worth trying. It was as though I had failed a test but with no suggestions on how to improve, when I felt like I had been trying my hardest.

We went on a joint mission to get Fin to put on weight. For my part, that meant ensuring he ate regular, varied meals, whilst continuing to breastfeed on demand. From Stuart's point of view that seemed to mean cakes and biscuits. He was only trying to meet the same ends as me, but perhaps going about it in a questionable manner.

This is part of why I find this weight obsessed situation worrying. It doesn't help to promote a healthy attitude to food. For instance, if I had been told that breast milk is more calorie and nutrient dense than solids, I would have focussed on breast milk more. There I was, trying to give more and more solid food to displace milk, when I should have been ensuring that Fin still got lots of breast milk! Had I relaxed and allowed Fin to feed himself, rather than panicking and trying to fill him with solid food, he might have fattened up a bit. In an 'obesity crisis', should we really be focussing on weight in babies in the way that we do, with mothers lacking information on what *should* make up a baby's diet?

I did my best. That's all mothers ever do really. We don't necessarily get it right but we try the best we can, through the guilt and worry. Now, I left the phase of exclusive breastfeeding and entered the uncharted territory of extended breastfeeding, however long that may be.

24

HOW LONG IS TOO LONG?

I'd decided I might breastfeed for around two years and, somehow, this made the concept of breastfeeding a two year old less weird to me. But I was aware, as every month passed, that we were something of a rarity. I only saw young babies being breastfed and when people talked about longer-term breastfeeding it seemed to be with some distaste.

Yet, it's largely in 'developed' countries that long-term breastfeeding has become uncommon, where feeding for six months is seen as more normal than six years. TV programmes and newspapers seem to love a story about a woman who has breastfed past infancy. It's seen as extreme.

But, biologically speaking, what should be the normal term of breastfeeding? Anthropologists have postulated natural weaning (and here I use the term to refer to the end of breastfeeding) is somewhere between two and seven years in humans.[1] There are different ways of estimating the natural term of weaning, such as studying traditional communities, examining dentition in fossils or comparing with primate behaviour, which is why the age is such a large range.

For instance, the !Kung wean between the age of two and three,[2] whereas Zulu mothers wean between twelve and eighteen months.[3] Although there is some cultural variability, most traditional societies wean by two to four years of age.[3] If the age of weaning is assumed to be when a baby quadruples its birth weight, then the child would be aged around two.[1] Perhaps the natural age of weaning is when the adult molars start to come in, around age six.[1] Anyway, we're so removed from what's biologically normal for our species that it's going to take a lot of science to figure things out.

Breastfeeding an older baby or toddler still has value. All the wonderful things about breast milk, its nutritional tailoring and immunological properties, they still hold true as the baby gets older.[4] But also, breastfeeding still performs that act of comfort, of checking in. If a child is upset, scared or there is some upheaval in their life, breastfeeding helps to provide them with security, in the arms of their mother. It's a repetitive, physical reminder of that parent-child bond.

For the mother, extended breastfeeding has links with reducing cancer[5] and osteoporosis.[6] For example, breastfeeding two babies for six months gives the same reduction in breast cancer risk as breastfeeding one baby for a year; the longer you breastfeed, the greater the effect.[7]

Some people could argue that breastfeeding an older child infantilises them. But yet, children have beds full of stuffed toys and so many of them 'have' to take their most beloved toy, or special blanket, or whatever comforting object they have, to their first day of school.[8] It should simply be a case of what suits the family and what is biologically normal for a child of that age.

Some argue that extended breastfeeding could lead to a clingy, dependent child. But many counter that a child who is given physical contact and attachment is far more likely to be independent.[9] Breastfeeding is one way of demonstrating this to a child. Children will become independent when they are developmentally ready to be – if you force them to stop breastfeeding at a young age then that's not really going to help. Being attached is not the same as being dependent.

Weaning can take place in different ways and for different reasons. One approach is child-led, whereby the child gradually consumes less breast milk until they no longer ask for it.[3] Some choose a mother-led approach, where the mother decides the end point before the child indicates signs of readiness.[3] This may be because she is going to work or because she has concerns about continuing to breastfeed, such as the child's growth.

Breastfeeding may also come to an end in the case of a nursing strike, which is when an infant suddenly refuses the breast.[3] A friend of mine's baby went on nursing strike because she had a cold and so struggled to breathe when she was feeding. Sometimes it's possible, with coaxing and nurturing, to get the child to breastfeed again, but sometimes it marks the end of the road, which was what happened in my friend's case. Finally, some babies wean in emergency situations, such as if the mother is seriously ill or dies, or if they are forcibly separated.[3]

For young babies who are weaned early, there could be issues surrounding their willingness to take a bottle that will need to be addressed. Also, a child younger than one will need formula milk. If they are older, whole cow's milk is a suitable substitute for formula.

Whatever the circumstances around the decision to wean, the ideal is to do so gradually. If weaning happens too abruptly, the mother can suffer from engorgement, blocked ducts and, potentially, mastitis, although expressing a little milk for comfort can help.[10] If instead breast milk is given in decreasing amounts the body can gradually adjust to the reduced demand.

After weaning, the body slows and stops milk production. Some women continue to produce milk for months afterwards,[11] something I found quite surprising.

For many mothers, complete weaning from the breast is an emotional time, perhaps in part due to fluctuating hormones.[12] It also marks the end of a significant part of their child's infancy and that can be very bittersweet.

So, how long should we be breastfeeding? How long is a piece of string? Breastfeed until you're both done with it. If you find yourself breastfeeding a walking, talking child, even one that goes to school, even though you're a rarity, you're actually very normal.

25

THE END OF THE ROAD

I loved my job (mostly). Since leaving university with a BSc in Marine Biology I've tried a few things, none of them being swanning about on a beach in a bikini looking at fish. Long story short, I sort of fell into being a secondary school teacher.

People told me I should be a teacher but I wasn't interested. It was only when I realised that I was always trying to teach people things (asked or not), such as karate, and diving, that I thought I should probably do something I naturally gravitated towards and enjoyed. The trouble was that I was distrustful of the profession; 'those that can, do; those that can't, teach'. I had had this firmly drummed into me by the world in general, so it took a while to realise that not only did I want to be a teacher, but also that it was a highly respectable and challenging career. It was what I should have been doing all along.

My teacher training was extremely hard. It transpires that 'those that can, do; those that can quickly, clearly and creatively under enormous pressure, teach.' I worked long, thankless hours planning, marking and organising and I threw myself into the intense challenge of teaching reluctant teenagers. This didn't change much when I qualified.

When I fell pregnant, I felt sad that I would be taking time out of a career that I had a lot of passion for. I felt like I was letting down my students. In fact, I'd tried to work my pregnancy around the school year; my due date was three weeks after the end of term, so I taught my kids right to the end. I was shattered, but it mattered.

I'd decided to take a whole year off. I wanted the maximum amount of time with my baby. Also, if I missed a whole academic year it would be much easier for me and my students than turning up midway through. Realistically, I would get few legitimate reasons in my life to skive off work for such an extended period of time without being fired, so I figured I ought to take advantage.

Once I had Finlay I couldn't wait to take him into work. Colleagues vied for cuddles and the pupils ran screaming towards me in the corridors and huddled around me like paparazzi. It made me feel missed at a time when I was struggling with feelings of isolation.

People told me to enjoy my maternity leave, it goes all too quickly. I honestly tried, but I often thought about my job. I still read my work emails and the Master's degree I was studying was in education. It helped me feel I wouldn't be totally useless on my return.

Still, as time wore on, I was glad I'd taken such a long maternity leave. With the extreme lack of sleep I doubt I could have functioned at work and, anyway, I wasn't ready to leave Fin. Just going out for a few hours had been hard enough. Much as I missed my job, being a mother had become everything to me.

I wanted to go back to work part-time but, for many reasons, my school refused. I was heartbroken; it was all part of my master plan. I knew how time-consuming full-time teaching is and it was hard to see how I could cope with that and a baby. But it wasn't to be.

I figured that, since I only had to be at school during school hours, I could fit the rest of my admin in at other times. That way, I could be with Fin for most of every evening. Besides, every six weeks I had school holidays when I could be with him all the time. I would have to work every time he slept, but it was a small price to pay to maximise my time with him. Sure, it would have been nice to work less hours, but it was either work full-time, or give up my job and try to find something suitable part-time, in a school where I would have to learn the ropes all over again. I loved Fin first and foremost, but I had to make a decision about how to balance that with my career.

We were lucky with our childcare situation. Stuart worked shifts, so a lot of the time he would be at home when I was at work. I knew I didn't need to worry about leaving Fin with his dad. When we were both at work, my in-laws, Angela and John, could look after him. I was so glad that Fin would always be with family if he couldn't be with me and that my return to work would help him grow close to his extended family.

Still, it was hard for me to accept having anybody but me looking after Fin, even his grandparents. Don't get me wrong, my in-laws are loving, kind people who adore their grandson. I knew he would be spoilt and given lots of attention and, of course, they had also raised two children of their own. But, they did things differently to me and my family. Not wrong, just different. As is seemingly the case with grandparents everywhere; they generally didn't do things the way I wanted. I'm a control-freak and my parenting was no different to every other aspect of my life. I wanted them to look after him in *my* way. It was hard to accept that wasn't going to happen.

One day, we were at my in-laws house. I was enjoying watching Angela and John play with Fin, but it tore at my heart. I was going to have to leave him. I had been there almost every moment since Fin was born. He was my baby; my moon, my stars; my reason for being. How could I leave him with other people, however wonderful they were and despite the fact he clearly loved them? I would miss him terribly and I was doing it all for what? Money and independence? Was it worth it?

I apprehensively set my date to return to work. I was looking forward to seeing everyone and getting a bit of my pre-baby identity back, but naturally I also worried about Fin. My thoughts turned to breastfeeding. By this point, he fed when he woke up in the morning, before his two naps, and at bedtime. I didn't know if I would need to express milk at work and how I would fit that into the school day. I worried that if Fin didn't get any milk during the day then he would make up for it at night and be more restless, returning to disrupted sleep.

I replenished the stocks of expressed milk in the freezer and took a little bag of Fin's clothes to his grandparents' house along with nappies and wipes. Angela and John stocked up on toys and bought a travel cot for Fin's naps. They were understandably excited, but their excitement was my impending doom.

Time waits for no woman and my maternity leave came to an end. On my first day back I was awoken at 4.30am needing a wee. I had a choice: I could get up, and probably wake Fin in the process, or I could lie awake and desperate in bed. While I lay pondering this dilemma I heard a little whimper from across the hall. I padded to Fin's room (via the bathroom) to be greeted by a beautiful smile from my baby boy.

I collected Fin from his bed and took him back to mine for a dozy feed. My mind was racing, going over the logistics of the day. Perhaps I should have been drinking him in, but breastfeeding isn't always as romantic as that. After twenty minutes of consternation I got up. Fin was dressed and breakfasted by six and I was good to go at seven.

Stuart took a picture, before I left, of Fin and I on this milestone day. I showered Fin in kisses and was shooed away by Stuart. I reluctantly got in the car, but I quickly forgot about reality as I sang at the top of my voice to the stereo on full blast, something I couldn't often do because of Fin's little ears.

I had an amazing day catching up with everybody. I had plenty of work to do, although no classes by some lucky chance. Before long my first day back was over and I was racing home to see my little boy. I had been inundated with texts and pictures all day to keep me informed of what was going on, but all the same, I couldn't wait to be home.

I walked in the door and rushed to pick Fin up. He turned to me for a kiss, paused, and said, 'Mum.' This might have been coincidence, since it was a sound he babbled, but I'm going to take it anyway. Fin and Stuart had spent a lovely day playing. My expressed milk had gone in a sippy cup at lunchtime and Fin had drifted off at nap-time sucking his dummy. A part of me wanted weeping and wailing but, obviously, it was better that he was happy.

As I settled back into work our childcare arrangements worked smoothly. Angela loved taking Fin to toddler groups and he seemed to be as happy with his grandparents as with me or Stuart. It was a huge relief.

It was hard being back at work. I felt like I was spinning too many plates in the air at once. At times I neglected to give attention to Fin, getting Stuart to take up the slack, and at other times I was slapdash about my job, and that isn't easy when your job involves the future lives of other people's children. I had to find the line, the acceptable point where I was doing adequately well by everyone.

Like any working mother, I was exhausted most of the time. I would get home from work and have to summon the energy to play with Fin. By the time he was settled in bed I was totally bushed, but I would then have to get the books out and do my admin. It was relentless; I was always either working or looking after Fin. My evenings were lost to paperwork and my dreams became nightmares about everything slipping into chaos.

Breastfeeding was becoming a smaller part of our lives. 'Two years and beyond' felt like a finishing line that I was determined to reach. I desperately wanted to last the distance, to be a 'good' statistic.

Nothing is straightforward. I started to find breastfeeding

uncomfortable, not painful like the early days, just sort of weird. I would impatiently look at my watch feeling frustrated that feeding was taking *this* long. The sensation of breastfeeding suddenly felt like fingers scraping down a blackboard. I had to grit my teeth to bear it. The sensation seemed to fluctuate depending on the time of the month. Sometimes breastfeeding felt normal, other times it made my skin crawl.

I think I was suffering from breastfeeding aversion (also known as breastfeeding agitation) which I suppose was linked to my hormones. It's a poorly understood phenomenon that makes breastfeeding feel unpleasant.[1] Sometimes, it's linked to a subsequent pregnancy but I knew this wasn't the case. I wonder whether the infrequency of my feeding Fin had an impact because I wasn't so 'used' to it. I don't know. Anyway, feeling 'weird' was never going to stop me. I was still aiming for two years and I am nothing if not determined.

However, since I'd returned to work our feeds had reduced down to just one before bed. Fin had got so used to managing without me while I was at work that he didn't ask any more and I never seemed to have the time to feed him before work.

When Fin was fourteen months old, breastfeeding became a wrestling match. Getting him to stay still and feed properly, it was like feeding an octopus. Fin's room had a wooden seagull suspended from the ceiling that flapped its wings when you pulled a cord. He had always ignored this...until now.

Feeding, once upon a time, used to end in Fin drifting off to sleep. Now I would dump him in his cot with his dummy, fed up of my nipples being dragged about by a fidgeting toddler, not that he seemed to care. I would kiss Fin goodnight and walk out and he would babble away to himself until he fell asleep. Breastfeeding no longer got him to sleep; it wasn't what it had been.

Fin didn't appear to be interested in breastfeeding; it was me that instigated it. I always offered, he never asked. Anyway, I didn't like breastfeeding any more. I had to ask myself why I was doing it.

I wanted to make it to two years but that seemed such a long way off. I didn't know what to do for the best. It seemed to me that it was a good opportunity to stop, since Fin seemed unlikely to notice the change. But, then, was I giving up too early because of convenience?

I made a decision. The time had come. It was the end of a significant period in our lives and it was sooner than I'd hoped. But breastfeeding is a two way relationship and I think both of us were done. I felt passionate about it in so many ways but I felt it was our time to stop.

It was hard to walk out of the room without feeding him that first time, my throat tight with emotion, but he was fine. He was fine the next night too, and the next. Fin never once pulled at my top or cried…nothing. He didn't miss it.

We had made it to a little over fifteen months. Whilst it wasn't as long as I'd hoped, it was a lot longer than the six months I had originally gritted my teeth and set my sights on. I knew I should feel proud. Instead of ending breastfeeding because I hated it I had stopped despite loving it. That seemed right somehow.

This journey that I had fought so hard for was over, just like that. It felt like I had only blinked since Fin had been born. We were no longer tied by this milky bond. I felt devastated and liberated in equal measure. Fin hadn't wept a tear or lost sleep over the end of this phase. I, on the other hand, had lost something that had made me the parent I was; that had defined me as a mother in so many ways.

I mourned those early days when things had been so needlessly difficult. I hadn't got to enjoy the heavenly aspects of early breastfeeding. There was only one way to change that, and to get the opportunity to experience the lovely moments again. Maybe I might even make it to two years.

If at first you don't succeed…

26

CONTRACEPTION AND BIRTH SPACING

I'd stopped breastfeeding before I thought seriously about having another baby. But I was aware that breastfeeding delayed the return of my periods, and so, fertility. Whilst I chose not to use breastfeeding as a form of contraception, some women do. Equally, for those that want to have another baby, breastfeeding is an important factor to consider.

The contraceptive effect of breastfeeding has been known about for a long time. As I've already discussed, historically, rich women would use wet nurses so that they were able to have plentiful babies to carry on their dynasties. For similar reasons slave women would have their babies taken away young, not only in the instance of being used as wet nurses, but when their owners wanted to breed more slaves.

Breastfeeding women often don't have periods (another benefit of breastfeeding) because feeding a baby regularly stops the body from ovulating by inhibiting the release of luteinising hormone, which, when it peaks, causes ovulation.[1] Really, this makes sense; if you have a young baby that is feeding regularly you can't easily invest in a new baby. Biology again is being clever by having a mechanism to protect new mothers from becoming pregnant when they have a very dependent baby. Female hormones are fascinating.

Some women use this contraceptive effect to their advantage. The lactational amenorrhea method (or LAM) as it's known is about 99% effective providing that certain criteria are met: the baby needs to be younger than six months, the woman's periods can't have returned and breastfeeding must be exclusive.[2] If these criteria aren't fulfilled then the effectiveness of the method is compromised.

One problem with this method is that you have no idea when your fertility has returned. Women can ovulate before their first period after birth; you can become pregnant without having had a single period.[3(pp238-239)] So you may be feeling confident that your fertility hasn't returned and breastfeeding is still working, only to find that you're pregnant. This is highly unlikely before six months though.

Anything that reduces suckling time at the breast reduces the contraceptive effect of breastfeeding.[4] For instance, using a dummy means that a baby is spending time sucking away from the breast. The use of formula also reduces time spent breastfeeding. Expressing milk, since it's less effective at stimulating milk production than a baby, can reduce the contraceptive effect of breastfeeding. Even sleep training a baby, so they go longer periods without breastfeeding, can have an impact. Essentially, the woman's body will act as if the baby is weaning and, therefore, less dependent. However, if nursing remains frequent then the contraceptive effect of breastfeeding remains high.

I certainly felt it was advisable to use other birth control methods; many women do. Once a baby is older than six months LAM becomes unreliable. But it's important to be aware that, if you are using hormonal contraceptive methods, some have an effect on milk supply because essentially you are upsetting the delicate hormonal balance in the body.[5] It's something that needs to be discussed with a doctor.

In some areas contraception isn't readily available; for example in parts of the world where medical facilities are inaccessible or expensive. Or it might be considered culturally inappropriate to use contraception. Some women have baby after baby, with little or no time to recover in between, and no choice to do otherwise. Sometimes that leads to women taking measures to end their pregnancies which aren't always safe. Of course, in some countries, childbirth is still a dangerous process which the mother, or the baby, doesn't always survive. If exclusive breastfeeding were more commonplace it could help many women to space out their births, reducing the number of times they need to risk going through childbirth or preventing them choosing a backstreet abortion.[6(p133)] In developing countries breastfeeding is often the only form of contraception available and, therefore, the only control women have over their pregnancies.[6(p133)] Breastfeeding information and support can save lives in deeper ways than you might think.

Breastfeeding women can get pregnant, especially as their babies get older and feed less frequently. Some women might struggle to fall pregnant while they are still breastfeeding an older child and so they might decide to cut down or stop feeds.[4(p170)] But then, it might be a signal that your body isn't ready for a new baby yet if you are still breastfeeding a dependent older child. Still, breastfeeding usually isn't harmful during pregnancy.[3(p210-233)] It's something unique to each woman's situation that she has to choose for herself.

My periods returned when Fin was six months old so I suppose, in theory, I could have had another baby at that point had I wanted one. I felt I had enough to deal with though.

If women do fall pregnant while breastfeeding, they can breastfeed through pregnancy, although some find it uncomfortable as their breasts become more tender.[7] This makes some women decide to wean the older baby. Milk supply can dip too, which some babies are fine with, whereas others decide to wean themselves.[7] There are amazing stories of older, talking, children noticing the change in milk and recognising that their mother is pregnant before she does.

If a woman breastfeeds through pregnancy she can continue breastfeeding after the baby is born, tandem feeding a newborn and a toddler. A woman's body is quite able to rise to this challenge too, in much the same way that it can ably feed twins. It's truly amazing.

My nana used to tell a story about feeding one of her babies and the older one 'having a little sip' too while she hid in a bush for privacy. It was always a story she told with a happy glint in her eye. I suppose, having weaned Fin, that it wasn't going to be a story I would get to tell, but I hoped at least to be able to have fed more than one baby. I wanted another go.

27

TAKE TWO⊙

Since Fin's birth I had insisted that I wasn't having any more children. Before, I'd wanted two children. Now, Fin was enough. Quite frankly, I was afraid, not just of birth but all the rest of it; the hardship of early parenting. Birth is such a fraction of time over the experience of motherhood; I could compartmentalise that. But I worried about the months that had followed Fin's birth; my difficulties breastfeeding and adjusting to motherhood. I didn't think I was able to go through it again, let alone actually *want* to.

I guess biological urges are strong. Just as life started getting easier, as Fin became less demanding, I started to crave a second baby. Through my fear I felt I could see her. You see, I knew she was a girl. She wasn't even a twinkle in her daddy's eye but I could see her face. I felt as though, if I didn't find her, I would spend my whole life looking. Of course, a boy would bring equal joy; I only needed to look at Fin to know that, but I felt a girl was next. So, as the memories of Fin's birth and early infancy faded I became more persuadable. A second baby would be such a blessing.

A companion for Fin, another special addition to the family...

Stuart, Fin and I went on holiday to America to visit family. In Stansted airport, at the bag-drop, Stuart says he saw a family. They had a little girl with pigtails, about two years old, following her bigger, school-age brother around. That night, Stuart told me, he dreamed about a little girl that looked like Fin but with long hair and a dress. He confessed to me how much he wanted to have a daughter, to have a family just like the one he had seen.

I found myself travelling home on the plane without the heavy load of drugs I normally need to even contemplate aviation because I had my suspicions I was harbouring a stowaway. Shortly after we returned, I felt those familiar early signs. My breasts hurt when I moved and I had a strange taste in my mouth so all my food tasted...*weird.* I felt a little out of it, mooning about something. This isn't unlike how I feel in the hormone addled days of pre-period blues, so I couldn't be sure.

Just a day or two short of when my period was due I was shopping in a chemist and I was drawn magnetically to the pregnancy test section. I started talking myself into it. I could get one ready for when I got home. I mean, it would save me another shopping trip.

I bought the test. I carried on shopping, but a large part of my subconscious was focussed on that little stick in my bag. I wandered over to the university library to pick up some books and thought I'd take the opportunity to visit the ladies' room; the toilets were nice there, unlike the gross ones in town that have to be locked at night to keep the drunks out.

In the stall, I put my bags on the floor, acutely aware of the contents. Again my subconscious started trying to talk me into taking the test. It would be a waste of urine really, wouldn't it? I ought to wait until I was home with Stuart, but he need never know. It was so early that it would surely be negative. I was just being curious...

Of course, I did it. I put the stick on the cistern while I gathered my things. It wasn't all significant and frightening like the first time, it was just something I happened to do while I was in the toilets; like putting on lip balm. I had just about finished gathering my belongings and rearranging my clothes as the allotted time ticked by. I glanced at the test, fully expecting it to be negative. There, right there, was the darkest line I had ever seen.

I froze. Obviously, it wasn't wholly unexpected, but I suddenly felt very guilty. I texted Stuart 'I have news'. He immediately phoned me.

'What? Is it what I think?' he said, as soon as I answered. Breathing quickly I answered, 'Yes. I'm so sorry I did it without you.'

'Don't be silly. See, we knew you were pregnant didn't we?!' he said, as I smiled in relief.

When I met my midwife for the first time I was all too aware of vehemently declaring to my last midwife, Jane, that I would never have another baby. She had knowingly smiled and told me she would see me in a year or two. Fortunately, I had a different midwife so I didn't have to worry that she would remember this exchange. My new midwife, Kate, who looked much younger than she professed to be, was absolutely lovely. She always kicked off her shoes as she came into my house, even though I'd told her she didn't need to. She was so friendly that I quickly grew to like her as much, if not more, than Jane.

On the day of the twenty-week scan my stomach was in knots because this was when we could confirm the gender. We had taken Fin, now two years old, in the hope that he would be excited to see the blurry black and white images of the sibling we had told him was coming. He, however, just wanted to play with the stickle bricks in the waiting room.

Stuart wrestled with an unwilling Finlay as the sonographer worked down the baby's body looking at each feature and checking that it was normal.

'Do you want to know the sex?' she asked when she reached the lower half of the body.

'Yes,' we both breathlessly replied. As the sonographer moved the probe it was quite clear to me what I could see and my heart skipped.

'It looks to me like you are having a girl!' The sonographer said.

'Thank God for that, we don't need any more children now,' said Stuart, picking up Fin under one arm and leaving to play with the stickle bricks.

As I watched her little legs being checked over a warm feeling spread over me. One of each gender! Although I liked the idea of having two boys, being brothers together, I knew that I would always crave having a girl so that I got to experience being a mother to both genders. Our little family was complete.

'Your placenta is a little low, let me measure it.' I was

woken from my reverie with a jolt. 'Yes, look it's very close to your cervix. It's nothing to worry about; chances are it'll move away as your womb grows. We'll need you to come back at thirty-two weeks to check its position.' With that matter of fact statement the scan ended.

I left with mixed feelings. I was delighted at the news I was having a girl. But the implications of a low-lying placenta, possibly requiring a caesarean, were worrying.[1] I felt the need for an intensive internet trawl to see what I could drag up. The sonographer had told me not to worry, but she didn't know me. The thing is, although this might not be something that would endanger our lives, it had wider implications for me because it could force me to have my baby in hospital.

I'd already decided on a home birth. My experiences first time around had left me with a rising panic any time I thought about being in a hospital again. Since I had ended up having a straightforward birth the first time I was still a suitable candidate for a home birth.

Our families tried to talk me out of it; I got warnings about haemorrhaging, the baby getting stuck, all sorts of things. My feeling was that the psychological damage from me being in hospital was also a sizeable risk and not one I was willing to take again unless I had to for the safety of my child. The far-reaching consequences of my treatment the first time around were not something I wished to repeat. I didn't want to revisit the scenes that had haunted me for quite some time.

I knew that being calm and focussed was key to an easy labour and I just couldn't visualise that happening in hospital. Anyway, I could get to hospital quickly enough in an ambulance if necessary. Realistically, it wasn't very different from the last time when I still needed to be transferred to hospital if anything serious happened, even though I was in a medical setting. It was merely a further five minute ambulance drive to the nearest hospital should the need arise.

Of course, when life is getting complicated, when you are busy and in a state of flux, what you should do is to add in an extra complicating factor. We got a dog. Without going into long-winded detail, the right dog came up at a time when we could take her.

We went to meet Dolly at the rehoming centre. She was young and trainable; ideal for a family with young children. She was a breed that we were familiar with since Stuart's family dog when we were first together was the same, a Staffordshire bull terrier crossed with a boxer. As soon as she saw us this bullet of a dog ran at us and lavished us with all the love she had.

A week later, I was driving home with a puppy in the boot. I took her into the house and she introduced herself to our home, dashing around it sniffing madly and rolling on all our carpets. Evidently, Dolly was home.

I was so busy balancing work and parenthood (and dog ownership) that I didn't have the time to think about my pregnancy. If anybody asked me, I didn't have the faintest idea of how many weeks pregnant I was.

I seemed to be keeping the weight off, which was no

surprise with running after Fin and walking Dolly. But I started to stiffen. I would feel achy around my pelvis when I got out of the car or stood up. Of course, with a growing baby bump and an active lifestyle, this was only to be expected. Or was it? When I walked it felt like the bones in my pelvis were grating and they seemed to almost get stuck. When I turned over in bed it hurt like I'd been kicked in the crotch.

Alarm bells rang. It sounded like something a friend had experienced in her second pregnancy called 'pelvic girdle pain' (PGP). As the name suggests, this is pain in the pelvic girdle. It's caused by the softening and stretching of the ligaments in your pelvis causing instability and pain.[2] Carrying around a heavy weight on top of that unstable base isn't pleasant. Fortunately, Kate quickly referred me to a physiotherapist.

I arrived at the slightly rundown local hospital, feeling incongruous as a huge staggering pregnant woman (I am too stubbornly cheap to pay for parking so, even though I was in agony, I parked far away and walked). I worried that the physiotherapist might tell me that it was just normal pain and I should stop my whingeing.

While I was daydreaming in reception, a busy looking, blonde lady came out and called my name. I followed her, painfully, through seemingly endless corridors to the treatment room. Although abrupt, she was kind and extremely gentle. She observed and felt my bone movement as I stood in various positions and decided that, yes, I did have PGP. She explained that one half of my pelvis was slipping down and then getting stuck, preventing the other side of my pelvis from articulating. Needless to say, this hurt. She taught me some exercises to help keep my pelvis aligned.

Although I could cope with the pain on a daily basis, I struggled at night. I needed a mountain of pillows to prop my body in a position where my hips didn't hurt. Typically, just as I got myself arranged I would need to go to the bathroom. I couldn't stay completely still all night and if I needed to turn over it would be excruciating. Sleep became fractured and the continual pain and fatigue was wearing.

A few weeks later I was at work and I needed to nip out of my classroom to grab some paperwork. I was rushing as much as a heavily pregnant woman with bad hips is able to rush (it's never a good idea to leave thirty-odd boys alone). Suddenly, I found myself slipping and a horrific shooting pain ran through my pelvis and up my bump. I saved myself from falling, but one leg had slid much too far in the splits position. I stood for a moment to regain my composure, hanging on to the wall for support. I saw the cause of my fall, a little puddle of water that had splashed on to the floor next to the water cooler that the students use.

In a school, an environment where there are normally people everywhere, there was suddenly nobody to be seen. This was a mixed blessing. On one hand, nobody had seen me slip. On the other, I was now in extreme pain and unable to move. I had a class waiting for me in my lab and I was stuck.

Clinging on to the wall I dragged myself round the corner to the staff workroom. I sat at my desk by the door, deciding what to do. There was nobody who could hear me if I shouted for help. I couldn't possibly leave my class unsupervised any longer so I decided to return to them and then get one of them to go for help. Gingerly, I walked back to my lab, wincing at every step. It was a year eleven boys' class (my school has single-sex teaching), not really the environment for me to break down in tears and beg for help. I wanted to retain my composure.

I called the pupils to order. This was normally a tiresome task, but I think they could see that I was on the verge of tears. I gave them an exercise to get on with. I didn't feel I could, after all, confess to one of them what had happened and I also had an overbearing urge to escape. Clinging on to the desks I made my way to the prep room next door where I knew a science technician would be. I felt the red rising in my cheeks as I left as quickly as the pain allowed.

As I gratefully lowered myself into a chair I started to explain to the technician what had happened. I felt so stupid. At that moment a teaching colleague also came in to ask for something, but seeing the state of me she stopped and enquired what was wrong. As soon as she realised my plight she kindly told me she would sort out my class and that, under no circumstances, was I to go back in there. The technician kindly gathered my bags from my lab and found me some painkillers.

I rang Stuart who instantly offered to come and pick me up. However, it would take him over an hour to get to me. I decided that if I could get to the car I could probably drive it, obviously checking first that I could depress the pedals and react as quickly as usual.

The only way out to the car park, that didn't involve stairs, was using the freight lift. Ah, the glamorous life of a pregnant woman. Utterly humiliated, I got in my car and checked whether I could use the pedals. As it transpired, the movements associated with driving caused me no pain whatsoever so, thankfully, I reached home quickly to take to my bed for the weekend. It taught me to take it easy, my poor hips couldn't stand it.

At thirty-two weeks, I went with my mum to the scan to check the position of my placenta. Stuart was working and wasn't overly interested in any more scans anyway. Since they hadn't scanned expectant mums when Mum was pregnant with me or Zack, it was an event she'd never witnessed so I thought she would like to take Stuart's place. As the image came up on the screen, Mum took in a breath.

'Wow, there she is!' she said. I had my mind on other things. I was, as before, unwilling to have a Caesarean-section, which there was a small chance of if my placenta was in a dangerous position. My tummy had survived my first pregnancy untouched by stretch marks or surgery scars and I intended to keep it that way.

'Let me measure the distance from the placenta to the cervix,' the sonographer said. I held my breath. 'Everything looks fine. There's no reason why you can't have a vaginal delivery.'

Relief flooded my body. I was going to have her at home. Now that the plan came into focus I realised I would have to experience birth again. My anxiety shifted from worrying about scars to worrying about pain.

One morning, a week before my due date, I started getting intense contractions. Not painful, but regular and strong.

They went on all day, leaving me thoroughly worn out. In the evening, convinced that tonight was the night, we phoned my mum and asked her to get Fin and Dolly; we figured this was better than calling her at two in the morning for an emergency pick up.

I hesitated; I didn't want to see Mum. In labour, I don't want anyone around. But Mum sensed this; she collected Fin and Dolly and left without speaking to me.

By midnight everything had stopped. I was mortified. We'd called Mum out for nothing. I felt I'd failed to produce the goods. I fell into a deep and frustrated sleep.

The next morning, Mum brought Fin home. He raced upstairs to the Moses basket beside my bed, peered in and burst into tears.

'Where's my sister, Mummy?' he asked. I choked back tears.

'She isn't ready yet. She'll be here soon though.' Fin was devastated. We'd been talking so much about the baby to prepare him that, understandably, he was disappointed. So was I.

We watched Fin in his first nativity play that day. He was a shepherd, but in the muddle we hadn't got him a costume. I threw my sequinned, silver snood over his head as he ran to join in. We giggled naughtily as he processed down the aisle, sequins glittering on his knitted, silver headscarf. I watched him gaze over the plastic dolly masquerading as Jesus. Where was his sister? She should be here by now. I sent a silent prayer for her to hurry up.

Christmas was careering towards us. It was impossible to

make plans without knowing when the baby was coming. I had crabbily told everyone that Christmas was cancelled as far as I was concerned; I was too fat, tired and angry. If I was still pregnant I would be in far too foul a mood to be festive; fielding benign and infuriating questions about my continued gestation. If the baby had been born I would be too tired and busy to undergo the stress of Christmas Day. If I was in labour then, obviously, I would be in no position to celebrate Christmas. Bah humbug!

On the evening of 22nd December the contractions started again. They were regular and pain started mounting. We phoned my mum, who, again, came straight away to pluck my sleeping son out of bed and remove Dolly. Mum laughed at me when she arrived because I was making last-minute Christmas presents out of felt from an amazing book that has patterns for gingerbread houses and Christmas tree decorations. After all, labour takes a long time; I needed something to do.

We started filling an inflatable birth pool in our living room. I had enjoyed the birth pool in my first labour and I didn't want to miss out just because I was having a home birth. I'd bought a second-hand, unused pool ready for the big day.

Filling it up had been something that worried us immensely. It would be no mean feat as, at the time, we had a cylinder central heating system. It would take four cylinders of hot water to fill the darn thing. That meant four lots of waiting for the cylinder to reheat. As we put the third batch of hot water in, my contractions disappeared and, at four in the morning, I crawled back into bed, despondent. I felt like a fool for calling Mum out again and spending hours filling an unused pool.

The next morning, 23rd December, was my due date so I had a midwife appointment. We'd asked Mum to keep Fin a while longer because we were shattered from the late night. There was no hiding the previous night's disappointment due to the hulking great birth pool that Kate had to edge round to sit on the sofa.

I explained to her that I was thoroughly fed up.

'Can't you do something, Kate? Can I have a stretch and sweep?'

'Not yet, it's still only your due date. Anyway, I wouldn't be surprised if things got moving along today. I'm not working later but I'll give you my mobile number in case something happens. I'd love to deliver this baby,' she smiled.

Despite Kate's reassurances I sulked. I was so fed up of being pregnant. I decided to take matters into my own hands.

'Let's go for a walk,' I announced.

'Oh?'

'Well, the boy is at Grandma's so we may as well make the most of it. Let's have lunch at that cafe on the cliffs. It must be about a three mile walk there and back? If that doesn't work nothing will.'

'What about your hips?' Stuart asked

'I'll manage.'

'What if you go into labour?' He looked unimpressed at my plan.

'We'll hammer on someone's door and make them drive me home. Don't worry, it probably won't work anyway, but I want cake.' I think Stuart knew better than to argue with a stubborn, angry and heavily pregnant woman.

We took an easy amble up to the cafe at the top of the cliffs, about a mile and a half from my house. I had my hips strapped up with a support band, although I knew I may still regret the walk later when I started to ache.

The walk did me good. It was a clear, winter's day, the grey sea meeting the white cliffs of Cap Blanc-Nez on the horizon. I felt the fog clear from my head and my mood begin to lift.

The cafe was quiet, with only an elderly couple sitting in one corner. The owner came to seat us, smiling.

'Goodness me, you must be due any minute!' she said.

'Yes, today,' I replied, grinning.

'She's been having contractions all night, but they stopped,' Stuart added. 'We took a walk to get things started again and thought we'd come here.'

Throwing her hands in the air, the proprietor exclaimed, 'You walked all that way? Oh my God!' She went to fetch our order quickly, probably to hasten our departure.

Looking out of the windows at the sea took the sting out of my lack of progress. After a pleasant lunch we started the slow walk back. As we walked I started to get niggling pains. By the time we were home they were gentle contractions. I decided to have a nap and when I woke up I was in labour. Definitely.

We put the last lot of the hot water into the birthing pool. I had been told to wait for a midwife before getting in, so I sat at the side, bouncing on my birthing ball, resting my head on the inflatable sides. We put on a film (*The King's Speech*) as a distraction from the steadily building waves of contractions.

Within an hour, Stuart had to rub my back every time a contraction came. Given my previous experience, I felt that, even though it was intense, it was nowhere near painful enough. My contractions were still about seven minutes apart so we held off phoning the midwife.

I was boiling hot so I stripped to a bikini. But, between contractions, I was shivering cold. It was hard to know what to do with myself. It was all too much. Stuart looked at me and I saw the realisation dawn in his eyes that I was no longer coping. Through the haze of pain I murmured, 'I can't do this any more.'

'Of course you can! But I'm going to ring Kate,' he said. Stuart turned off the TV and tried to call Kate's mobile, but there was no answer. He rang the hospital and got put through to the on-call midwife who said she would be over as soon as possible. Unbeknown to me, she could hear me groaning and knew with her midwife spidey-sense that I didn't have long to go, so she rang a colleague to see if they could get to me quicker.

Stuart came back to my side and, by this time, I was in a state. The contractions weren't fading. Ordinarily, the pain subsides so you get a chance in between to lie still and pray it will be over soon. But the pain wouldn't stop fizzing in my back and I was crying, desperate for relief.

I was vaguely aware of Stuart's phone ringing again. It was the midwife asking for directions. I was pleading for her to hurry up but could tell from the directions Stuart was giving her that she was still at least ten minutes away.

I needed to stand to take the pressure off my back. As I stood I was wracked with a powerful contraction that forced me to push down with such strength it took my breath away.

I roared with the pain of it.

'She's coming!' I screamed. As I lapsed into sobs, Stuart put a hand on my shoulder saying, 'Yes, she's coming. The midwife will be here any minute.'

'Not the midwife!' I cried through gritted teeth as another powerful wave hit me. I collapsed to the floor and clawed at my underwear. At this point Stuart saw the 'she' I was referring to.

28

THE CHRISTMAS BABY

'Oh my God, keep her in!' Stuart cried as he prodded at his mobile frantically. Dialling 999, he simultaneously shoved an old sheet under me.

All I remember was screaming at the top of my lungs as the baby was born, with Stuart keeping up a running commentary to the dispatcher on the phone. As my daughter's body slid into Stuart's arms my waters exploded all over his jumper. He lifted her on to my chest as I lay shivering with shock. He then wrapped us both in old sheets as I held her little naked body to my skin. She had jet black hair and the most beautiful little rosebud mouth.

The baby cried so I followed my instincts. I held her to my breast and, gazing at me with deep blue eyes she opened her mouth wide and started to feed like an old pro; that familiar feeling making me gasp in recollection. I couldn't quite take it all in; the birth had been so easy and she was so unbelievably beautiful, I wanted to remember how she looked in that moment forever. I tried to burn it on my memory.

Stuart was still on the phone to the dispatcher, a distant buzz in the background as her little face filled my entire world.

'Hello Mae,' I said. We'd chosen her name when we were expecting Fin. I've always loved words with 'ae' in them.

We were interrupted by a hammering at the door. Stuart went to answer and returned with a midwife and two paramedics. Suddenly, there was chaos and I was aware of the stupid position I had ended up in, lying between a sofa and the birth pool, fairly inaccessible by anyone's standards. I pulled the sheet over my legs to cover my dignity from the two male paramedics.

The midwife briefly, and discretely, checked me over, before there was another knock at the door signalling the arrival of a second midwife. My room was now ridiculously crowded with six adults, a baby and a huge birth pool.

The midwives decided I needed to be on the sofa to deliver the placenta, so somebody threw a shower curtain over it (we'd bought shower curtains to act as waterproof sheets should we need them) and the midwives helped me up while Stuart had his first cuddle with Mae. It was agony to move but, with their help, I managed to haul myself up. I noticed, as this happened, that one of the paramedics, casting around for something to do, saw my glasses on the sofa and picked them up and put them on the bookcase. This was the only thing these poor men did in the whole proceedings.

Lying on the sofa I latched Mae back on and fed her as her cord gradually stopped pulsing and the blood stopped flowing between us. I hadn't been given the choice to do this with Fin; the cord was cut instantly without questions. However, delayed cord clamping, to allow placental blood to transfer to the baby and prevent anaemia, had become more common.[1] Stuart was called over to cut the cord, which, this being his second time, he did nonchalantly.

Once it was established that I was not going to haemorrhage, the paramedics decided their presence was unnecessary and they sloped off. I later heard my own birth story back from a friend of one of those paramedics. Not that I mind, my emergency birth was the talk of the village anyway, but it made me laugh when I was told my own story.

I was covered in blood, sweat and goodness knows what else so the midwife suggested that I got into the birthing pool for a wash. She grabbed the thermometer that was floating about on the surface, only to find that it was too cold. So, after the stress of choosing the damn thing, the money spent on it, the day filling it and the wasted gas heating it, I never got to even put so much as a toe in it.

The midwives wanted to weigh Mae but she was hanging on to my breast with a determined ferocity. Eventually, despite the midwives' protestations to let me carry on, I stuck my pinkie finger in her mouth, broke the suction and levered her off, as she desperately reached out and nuzzled for more. The midwives weighed her at a healthy 7lb 6oz.

We decided this was an opportune moment to dress her and Stuart was chosen for the job. He started casting about the room looking for the clothes. I sighed; again he'd paid no attention when I told him where everything was. Once my bags had been found, Mae was put into the same first outfit that her brother had worn: a white vest, babygro and hat. It's an outfit I will always treasure.

The first midwife left, leaving just me, the baby, Stuart and midwife number two who started to help Stuart with the clean-up operation as I lay feeding my little girl (Mae had got straight back to it as soon as she was handed to me). Eventually, the sucking slowed and Mae's eyes closed, her body relaxing into sleep.

Stuart took Mae and the midwife offered to run me a bath. That felt like luxury: somebody else running me a bath in my own house, even thoughtfully adding a little bubble bath. She came back down to help me up the stairs, leaving me at the door.

'I'll give you some privacy. I'll be here at the top of the stairs in case you feel light-headed or anything. Just call and I'll come,' she said. I closed the door, looking around gratefully at my own, clean bathroom with all my own lotions and potions. No cracks, no ground in grime; it was so different from the last time.

I was aware, from the soreness down below (and having been told by the midwives), that I had torn again, but not so badly as before. I gingerly undressed and climbed into the bath. The water was bliss for my aching muscles and, although it stung, it was bearable. I lay there, without the pressure of imminent visitors, unworried by how long I had or whether someone could walk in. But yet, I had the security of the midwife still close at hand, doing her paperwork at the top of my stairs.

Soon I wanted to get back to Mae so I got out of the bath and wrapped my towel around me. I realised that my maternity sanitary towels were in another room. I considered calling the midwife and asking her to get them, but on hearing me get out of the bath she'd scurried downstairs to maintain my privacy. I walked across the landing and sorted myself out. But, as I turned back to the bathroom, I saw a trail of blood marking my journey. I sighed.

'Are you OK?' the midwife called.

'Yes,' I replied, getting a cloth and bending to clear up the blood. The room swam. I steadied myself with a hand on the wall, deciding whether to call out. The room slowed to its normal, static position so I gingerly cleared up the spots, taking my time to prevent the room spinning again.

I descended the stairs and gathered Mae back up. Stuart scrubbed the living room carpet (the shower curtain and sheets on the floor hadn't completely protected my cream carpet) and made tea for the midwife, while she and I chatted. She had to stay for two hours to make sure I was OK. Taking no chances this time, I made sure to tell her that I'd felt light-headed. She reassured me, but told me to take it easy.

I felt totally comfortable with this midwife, a complete contrast to my first experience. She was good at making herself at home and acting like an old friend. She was unobtrusive; sensitive as to when to be quiet and when to be companionable. She made me feel like I had her time and her attention. She also seemed to be an expert at removing blood stains, which I suppose, as a midwife that attends home births, you need to be. When the end of her two hour stint ticked round she left, saying what a wonderful birth it had been (not that she'd been there, which made us laugh).

Stuart got me a bowl of cereal since I was now ravenous, and turned the movie back on. The pool stood, unused and full in front of me. It was so surreal. It was as if time had frozen a few hours before and a baby had been just plopped into our arms. Life was exactly the same, but not the same. We gazed at the warm, sleeping bundle in my arms. Everything had been so *easy*. I had felt safe, despite the lack of professionals present and the suddenness of the whole thing. Once the midwives had arrived, I'd felt so cared for and supported. It had been a truly wonderful experience.

We were soon on the phone and Facebook. Immediately, responses of disbelief rained in: 'No midwife? Delivered by daddy? At home? Weren't you scared? Was it planned?' We smiled, smugly, and took ourselves off to bed.

I slept soundly, but each time Mae's little body started to wriggle next to me I awoke. There was no question about co-sleeping this time, we just did it. She fed around every two or three hours like a dream. At about two in the morning those big blue eyes were wide open, full of wonderment and wakefulness. I too was awake, drinking in her every clumsy movement and snuffly breath. I could remember lying awake with Fin in the same way when he first came home. Awake together while the world slept, and so in love.

The next day, Mum brought Fin and Dolly home to us. I had been anxious about Fin's return: it was a moment I'd been worrying about ever since I'd found out I was pregnant. How was my baby boy going to take meeting his little sister? I'd bought him a present from Mae; some trains for his train set. It's a crazy thing, pretending that this newborn baby had been shopping. But kids are gullible, I suppose, and I thought it might ease the transition.

Fin ran in. I was holding Mae in my arms, which I'd been planning not to do because I didn't want him to feel replaced, but I hadn't had time to put her down. Fin threw something red on to my lap and then ran to his train set, assuming his usual position. I looked down at the toy ladybird he had thrown at Mae, disinterested though he seemed.

'He picked it out himself, he was so excited to get something for her; quite the proud big brother,' Mum said. I called Fin over and gave him his present, which he opened immediately. I asked if he would like to hold his new sister. Fin shook his head and headed back to his trains with his new acquisition.

Angela and John arrived soon after and all the grandparents were vying for baby cuddles. It was lovely having my family about me with Mae sleeping in my arms and Fin playing at my feet. Things were a bit cramped, though, since there was still an enormous birthing pool in the centre of the room. It was decided that the visitors should make themselves useful.

A hose was set up to siphon out the water from the pool and, as the level dropped, it was also gradually deflated. When it had been emptied enough to be lifted, John and Stuart carried it out to the garden and dumped the remainder of the water in the flower beds. As they lifted the pool they revealed a puddle of blood that had been trapped underneath. I felt my face flush; my whole family could see it. Everybody was matter of fact but I was mortified even though, of course, we couldn't have cleaned up under a, seemingly, million ton pool.

I was stuck under a breastfeeding baby so I couldn't leap up and deal with the mess myself. Fortunately, the grandmothers sprang to action. They picked up the shower curtain that was acting as a waterproof sheet under the pool, one at each end. Blood started dripping on to the floor as the pair of them dithered about where to take it until Stuart came in and ushered them outside. That image of them looking panicked, holding a shower curtain with a pool of day old birth blood dripping on the floor, is etched into my memory for life.

After the clean-up operation everybody left and, for the first time, we were just us, a complete family unit. Of course, this being Christmas Eve, before Finlay retired for the night he put out mince pies, a glass of milk and babbled about his presents. We simply couldn't have been happier.

Christmas Day dawned. Fin ran into our room brandishing his stocking and we produced one for Mae which he delightedly 'helped' her with. This soothed Fin's excitement sufficiently for us to persuade him to wait for the rest of his gifts. Zack was staying at our mum's house and they would be heading over later so we wanted to wait for them. To pass the time we decided to head to church.

We'd never left the house with two children before. It's not very easy to do. Firstly, I was desperately trying to squeeze into some item of clothing that didn't resemble a sack. We also had to fill Fin's change bag with bits for Mae. Flustered, we ran out of the door with Mae in Stuart's arms and Fin in his pushchair. We were running late so we hastened as much as we could. The walk was surprisingly easy given that it was only about thirty hours since I had given birth. This would have been unthinkable last time.

As we neared the church the bells stopped ringing, signalling that we were late. We snuck through the door as quietly as we could, trying to slink to our usual seats unnoticed, but we were spied by the vicar.

'Amen.' (Or I assume words to that effect.) 'Oh my goodness, you've had the baby! Please come and show her off!'

Red faced, I crept to the front with my tiny bundle in my arms to the sound of applause and 'ahhhs'. Stuart and Fin sidled over to our usual seats.

'So, when was she born?' the vicar asked, beaming,

'Just over twenty-four hours ago, on the 23rd,' I said. There was more applause and an intake of breath.

'Did you get the home birth you wanted?' she asked. Before I could answer a voice came from the pews.

'Well, actually, I delivered her!'

'Oh my goodness, well come up here!' Stuart strode to the front of the church as I tried to disappear. He proceeded to give a blow by blow account (including waters bursting all over him and blood everywhere, like a Tarantino film) as I willed him to stop before I went a brighter shade of red. Nonetheless, the church members were delighted with the birth of a real baby at Christmas time and Stuart was brimming with pride.

Despite my embarrassment, I did feel special. To this day, the congregation still talks about the day that we brought our Christmas baby. Mae may not have been born on Christmas Day, but she still made Christmas memorable for a lot of people.

Of course, having just given birth, I was in no state to organise a Christmas celebration but I was fortunate enough to have family rally round. Mum and Zack looked after us, cooked the dinner and generally prevented me from needing to move. Then, after they had helped put the kids to bed, they went back to Mum's house to give us some peace.

People had all been so wonderful. From health professionals, to family, to complete strangers, everybody had made Mae's arrival so special. What could have been a frightening, sudden birth had, instead, been a wonderful experience thanks to the care and support we received. Christmas is a time for familial love and I don't think I ever have, or ever will, feel more Christmassy than I did that day.

29

BABYWEARING

Now that I had two children I had to find some way to deal with a toddler whilst also holding a baby in my arms. Children have a tendency to need things simultaneously, just to be awkward.

Before I had babies I thought that you fed them, changed their nappies and then put them down in a cot or on a play mat. If you needed to transport them anywhere, they went in a pram. Simple! I didn't realise that babies expect to be carried around all day, being the primal little primates that they are.

Fin wanted to be held all the time. Mae turned out to be much the same. This time around, though, I knew it was normal and, rather than trying to train my baby out of it, I indulged it. I looked for coping mechanisms to manage a tiny, clingy baby and a demanding toddler. The solution came in babywearing, which is a term that refers to carrying your baby in some kind of carrier.

As far as a baby is concerned, as soon as you put them down they are in dire peril. They feel safe in their parents' arms, protected from wolves and suchlike. They are unaware of the thousands of years of social changes that have brought us to the world of cots and pushchairs. A rocking cradle or jiggled pram simulates the motion that a parent makes when they hold their baby, it calms them down. A baby carrier can do this more convincingly.

There are various kinds of carrier. Different carriers are designed to suit different body types or needs and it's up to individual taste or lifestyle as to which is the most suitable. It can seem a bit overwhelming when you have so much choice but there is lots of online support and some areas have sling libraries where you can try and borrow different styles.

A wrap is a long piece of stretchy or woven fabric that is tied around the body in various different ways to secure the baby to your front or back.[1(pp122-160)] These might look daunting but they're actually fairly simple to master. There are Mei Tais, an Asian style of carrier, that consist of an oblong of fabric that the baby sits in and four straps which tie around the parent.[1(p167)] Structured carriers are similar to Mei Tais but are more padded and have buckles.[1(pp116-120)] Ring slings are a long piece of fabric with a ring on one end which can be quickly thrown on and tightened around the baby.[1(p165)] Other carriers exist but some are, perhaps, less ideal ergonomically.

A baby carrier enables the wearer to go about much of normal daily life with a content, snuggled up baby secured to their body. Baby carriers mimic the motion that a baby would be familiar with from being in the womb; they can still experience the natural walking gait and body sounds of a parent.[2] Some baby carriers allow easy access to the breast so babies can be nursed while the mother gets on with her day,[3(pp108-111)] snuggled close to help produce milk-making hormones. Babies can observe the world from a safe place, learning about how their parents go about their normal days. Babywearing means hands are free for any task (cleaning, gardening, cooking etc). For many women it's the ticket to getting their life 'back' rather than being stuck holding a needy baby.

Babywearing also provides a way for fathers to get involved in parenting in a close, attachment style way. Whereas breastfeeding can cause some tension for a father who wants to be hands-on, babywearing is something anybody can enjoy.

Often we think of traditional cultures when we think about carrying babies: perhaps women in Africa carrying their babies on their backs while they work and then swinging them round for a feed; or an Asian woman smiling with a baby in a Mai Tei on her back. But the truth is that examples exist all over the world. For example, in the UK, Welsh women traditionally carried babies in nursing shawls.[3(p20)]

Some traditional carriers are more unusual, such as the Bilum from Papua New Guinea, which is like a large mesh bag suspended from the forehead.[4] Navajo cradleboards consist of two pieces of wood, often with a footrest and a piece of wood to support a sun shade, that the baby is strapped to for much of the day.[5] The latter has been subject to research concerning an increased chance of hip dysplasia due to the baby's legs being straightened rather than supported in the hip tuck position that other carriers promote.[6]

In many countries, baby carrying has fallen out of popularity in favour of prams and pushchairs. I was never one of those mums who drooled over beautiful prams. My mum dragged me to the pushchair section at a baby show when I was pregnant with Fin and I reluctantly agreed to look at them but refused to buy one full price. I later bought a second-hand one that I didn't hate too much. I found them cumbersome and annoying to navigate around shops (it took me eight attempts to pass my driving test – I wasn't much better with a pram!). Neither of my children took to them when they were little and they would scream their heads off, not be eased to sleep (I promise it wasn't because of my steering). A carrier, on the other hand, was pretty much guaranteed to calm a fractious baby. As a good friend of mine says 'carriers come with magic, sleepy dust'.

But still, prams and pushchairs suit lots of people. In the eighteenth century the Duke of Devonshire had a carriage designed for his children that could be pulled by miniature horses or goats[7]…and, in some ways, I wish this still existed. Times moved on and, in 1852, the first patent for the 'perambulator' was filed by Charles Burton (now with a handle so it could be pushed).[7] Prams subsequently became extremely popular with Queen Victoria making them the height of fashion.[8] Today, they remain an item of style; the pram that Princess Charlotte was wheeled to her christening in (previously used by the Queen to push Prince Andrew) was the talk of the tabloids. They range from inexpensive to extremely pricey. Designs vary from prams where the baby lays flat to pushchairs that face their parents or face forwards to double pushchairs and goodness knows what else. Lots of people love them. I don't; I use them when it suits my needs, but I like to babywear more.

The first baby carrier I bought was poorly designed. When I had Fin the most fashionable styles seemed to be structured carriers where the baby faces forwards and basically dangles from its crotch, like in the film *The Hangover*. Things have moved on and safer, more ergonomic carriers are much more common.

The principle of a good carrier is that the baby sits with their whole bottom supported from knee to knee in an 'M' shape, either facing the parent or on their back.[1(p112)] Carriers also get expensive; the most beautiful designs can cost a pretty penny, but they generally hold their value for resale. A market has sprung up selling cheap imports that haven't been tested to the same rigorous standards to ensure babies are safe, so it's important to buy from reputable retailers or hire from somebody who knows what they're doing.

If you use a baby carrier there is a set of guidelines to ensure that the baby is as safe as possible, remembered through the acronym 'TICKS'.[3(p160)] It should be *tight*, the baby should be *in view* and *close* enough to kiss, you should *keep* the baby's chin off their chest and the back should be *supported*. If a baby carrier is used safely then it is an amazing way to transport your baby.

Babywearing makes me think about the concept of kangaroo care. Developed in Colombia, Kangaroo care is where premature babies are laid skin-to-skin on their parent's chest, covered with a blanket, as often as possible.[9]It's been found to reduce mortality and help babies to regulate their tiny, delicate bodies.[10] Rather than being in an incubator, often leaving their parents feeling very impotent, kangaroo care allows parents to bond with their babies and do something very real for their health. Being physically present, holding your baby, actually helps them to thrive.

To me, babywearing combines lots of ideas. It's a tool to cope with a dependent baby, enabling a mother to get on with her day or look after an older child. It's a way to transport a child that keeps them close so that you can communicate with them and respond to them, even breastfeed them. It's a way to have more physical closeness in an age where humans seem to be becoming more isolated. I used baby carriers a little with Fin, but now I had another baby they were indispensable.

30

COMPLETION?

We had everything we ever wanted; our family was complete. It wasn't easy, of course; there were new challenges to face. But I felt strong, confident and prepared this time.

Now, the thing about having a baby at home is that, other than the initial checks the midwife carries out, everything else has to be done at a hospital or doctor's surgery. Having a baby at Christmas means that a lot of places have closed for the holidays. We were told Mae had to be checked by a paediatrician within seventy-two hours of her birth. However, since she was evidently perfectly healthy it was put off until after Boxing Day. It was a wholly less stressful affair than waiting on a doctor to appear when they had time.

The midwife, Kate, kept a watchful eye on us over Christmas. It turned out that, during Mae's birth, Kate hadn't answered the phone because she'd had a car accident. Fortunately, nobody was hurt. Kate seemed genuinely disappointed she hadn't been a part of the birth and was now busily ensuring that Mae was a picture of health. All too soon our time was up. I was sad to be discharged from her care, having really bonded with her.

A few days in, my nipples started to feel bruised. I was worried in case it was a recurrence of my experiences the first time. This time I was proactive and texted the lady who now ran my local breastfeeding support group (Ruth had moved on) to ask what I should do. Just a few hours later a handful of nipple balm samples were pushed through my letterbox, along with some tips on positioning and attachment. It's funny how asking for help works when you ask helpful people.

It did the trick and I was comfortable breastfeeding in no time. I felt good too; I was up and about in a matter of days; not because I'd forced myself but because I wanted to be.

Soon, the fateful day came when Stuart had to go back to work. We had been lucky that Mae's birth fell over a bank holiday, meaning Stuart's paid paternity leave kicked in a bit later. But still, time does insist on rattling by. Up until this point, I'd looked after Mae while Stuart looked after Fin. But now what? How on earth was I going to look after two young children? When I had Fin I had been anxious about how I would manage alone. This time I didn't need the emotional backup so much, but the logistics of two children and one parent were terrifying.

I quickly discovered how well I could multitask whilst feeding. For instance, I could sit cross-legged on the floor playing with Fin's wooden trains with one knee raised to support Mae's body while she happily sucked away. This was rather lovely since in pregnancy I had continually frustrated Fin with my inability to sit on the floor, especially since I had been in so much pain with PGP. I also found I could walk around feeding Mae, holding her with one arm while using the other to deal with Fin. I could get through the day, feeding on the fly.

With Fin, breastfeeding had been all-consuming. I had been able to focus entirely on feeding the baby and relax while I did so. But now, a peaceful feed was out of the question and there was no chance of me quietly settling Mae into her Moses basket. I couldn't disappear into Mae's room for half an hour to get her settled because I had to supervise Fin, but I also couldn't play loud games while trying to get a small baby to sleep.

I remembered seeing a stretchy wrap demonstrated at breastfeeding group when Fin was about a year old. I regretted my choice of carrier with Fin since it wasn't particularly comfortable for me and wasn't ergonomically designed for him. I realised babywearing would be the way forward with two children. I could carry Mae in the sling and have both arms and legs free to do whatever I needed to do while she slept. This time I wanted to try a stretchy wrap.

Mae lived in her wrap for the first few months of her life. Being able to let her sleep while I walked Fin to nursery, played with him, or while I did housework was an absolute godsend. Whilst this five metre strip of fabric initially looked scary it turned out to be a breeze to use and was essential to my everyday life.

It was around this time that I submitted the dissertation for my Master's degree. This beast had taken me a year to write and the final finishing touches were made with newborn Mae snuggled in a wrap breastfeeding, at the university. At least I wouldn't have to struggle to lectures, leaving a baby behind. It was all done.

For my dissertation I'd researched the teaching of breastfeeding in schools. Given my experience of going from complete ignorance to struggling to breastfeed I felt that, rather than learning about breastfeeding at antenatal classes (if you're lucky), education should begin at school. It's a wonder that a physical process that defines us as mammals is largely ignored in schools. If school is a system to prepare children for adulthood it seems pretty important to explain how babies are fed. I teach children about sex, STIs, the menstrual cycle and pregnancy. Why does it stop there?

Writing a dissertation on this subject was the perfect culmination of studies that had taken place through my two pregnancies and early parenting experiences. My children are both in the picture of me 'in my funny hat' (as Fin would call it) because they were a big part of me earning that degree.

I soon realised that when I had been worn out, tired and run off my feet with one child, I hadn't known I was born! With one baby, after a bad night I only had to last until his nap-time and then I could usually get in a quick snooze. But the chances of two children being asleep at the same time were slim. Thank goodness for nursery! For two mornings a week I got to recharge my batteries while Fin went and wore himself out.

While I was more tired as a mum of two, I wasn't on the same emotional roller coaster. I didn't continually second guess myself, or live in perpetual guilt. I didn't fret about everything being perfect. I was exhausted, but I was fine. I couldn't have said I was fine the first time.

It wasn't easy, though. I was run ragged trying to balance entertaining Fin with meeting Mae's needs. Still, I was far from bored so I didn't have the time to wallow in self-doubt or obsess about how tired I was. Plus, I had a little two-year-old to chat to so I wasn't lonely either. I quickly fell into a routine of attending children's groups along with the daily rhythms of eating, sleeping and playing.

Naturally, there were times when I felt like I barely spoke to grown-ups and days when I didn't leave the house. However, I found the solution was to ensure I got at least ten minutes of head space a day. That might sound a bit crazy; ten minutes isn't much. But it gave me time when I wasn't trying to ensure that both of their needs were met, tracking where they both were, or considering my next move when the current activity ran out.

I found that a short dog walk (leaving the kids with Stuart) was enough to keep my sanity. Where I had been torn two ways after having Fin, I was now meeting the needs of three people; I had to get breaks. I couldn't get more than ten minutes since Mae wouldn't tolerate being parted from me for long. But those few minutes helped me to survive.

When Mae was three months old my mum had an operation

on her foot. Since Mum was going to be bed-bound she came to stay with us. She felt terrible because the timing was bad with us having a young baby, but it couldn't be helped. I was going to have to cook for her, help her to and from the toilet and look after her Yorkshire terrier, Riley. But, of course, family is family and so none of this mattered. We would find a way to manage.

The day of the surgery dawned and Stuart (instructed to be nice since Mum was anxious) took her to the hospital. I'd prepared Fin, explaining that Grandma was having her foot fixed and would have a big bandage.

Mum arrived at my house in the afternoon with an enormous cast and seeming rather chipper. She got herself up the stairs to her room by shuffling up on her bottom like a toddler might and seemed rather pleased with herself for being so brave. However, as the anaesthetic started to wear off she was clearly in more pain. Mum didn't want to be any trouble, but I tried my best to pop into her room regularly to offer her anything that would provide relief.

Mum recovered quickly but was constantly worried about being a burden. She wouldn't believe it, but she was quite the reverse, she was extremely useful. When I had a shower, Mum would hold Mae and try to stop her from crying (previously Mae would just cry through my showers on the floor of the bathroom). As Mae got more used to Grandma, I was able to wash my hair, dry my hair and get dressed without any screaming, which was quite a treat! Mum would also play with Fin or let him watch TV with her when I needed a moment away from him. I was so used to struggling single-handed while Stuart was at work that it was heavenly to have somebody to entertain the kids for a moment.

Help is so valuable. Mothers often have to manage alone much of the time. Generally, husbands are out for much of the day and, since we no longer (in my culture) live in extended family groups, mums can become very isolated. Some company and an extra pair of hands makes all the difference. If you have a friend with young children, offer to watch the kids for ten minutes. Your offer will be invaluable.

Anyway, we felt it important that Mum got out of the house so she'd hired a wheelchair. For our first undertaking, I helped her bump down the stairs on her bottom (no mean feat in itself) and then out to the wheelchair by the front door. Fin climbed up on to her lap and I strapped Mae to my front in her carrier.

We walked to the play-park, normally a five minute stroll from my house. By the time we were halfway there we were in fits of laughter because of the sight we presented, little old five foot three me, pushing my mother and son in a wheelchair, with a baby strapped to my front. In the weeks that followed I often took Riley too. It wasn't good for my back, but it was funny. I was the epitome of multitasking mum and, thanks to an amused passing stranger; I have the pictures to prove it.

Mum went back home after two weeks and I missed her terribly. Although I had less to do, I was, once again, left in sole daytime care of the kids with no adult to talk to. Twice a week, for the next six weeks, I popped to Mum's house to do jobs for her and keep her company as her mobility improved. While she thanked me endlessly for dragging out my young family to help her, I don't think she ever really saw how much it meant to me to spend time with her.

I felt it was time to get more involved in the world of breastfeeding. I'd finished my Master's degree and was eager to do more learning. It was time to 'pay it forward' by volunteering with my local breastfeeding support group.

Having faced breastfeeding challenges myself I could see how easy it was for things to go badly and I knew how much it hurt physically and emotionally. I wanted to help and was only too glad if people asked me questions. I wanted to tell people what I had been through so they could benefit from my experiences, to ensure the same thing didn't happen to them.

When Fin was little I'd become involved in antenatal breastfeeding workshops. They were run by Ruth, the midwife who ran the support group. When she needed mums to talk at her workshops she would use women from the breastfeeding group. I yearned to be the 'example' mum. On the one hand, I didn't want to scare a load of pregnant mums with my horror stories but, on the other, I felt I had a lot of useful experience to share. My story was real, and could demonstrate the benefits of perseverance and the importance of asking for help when needed. I could be the example of what *not* to do. I volunteered immediately when the offer came up. I was apprehensive; I knew that these kinds of encounters could be life-changing for expectant mothers.

On the day of the workshop I arrived with Fin and entered the very same room that my workshop had been held in more than a year previously. There was a small group of five mums-to-be. Three of us were volunteering, one with a month-old baby, one with a three-month old, and me with my now nine-month old. As I chatted away, I began to feel confident that I made the right decision to go along. I talked about how I should have asked for help, instead of soldiering on like a stubborn old mule, and how breastfeeding could still become wonderful despite a rocky start.

I felt passionate about passing on my newly-acquired knowledge and experience to a group of women who could, hopefully, be more successful in their quest than I, but who might also go on to love breastfeeding just as much as I had. I hoped something I said would make someone else's life a bit easier; that it would encourage somebody to ask for help or make them realise that it was OK not to love every moment of breastfeeding.

Sometime later, I went along to breastfeeding group as usual. I was chatting to a new mum, trying to make her feel welcome in her first visit to the group. It transpired that she had been one of the ladies in that workshop and she remembered some of the things I'd said and had found them useful. I felt so proud. I had done my 'good thing' on that day. I hadn't been the black cloud of depression over proceedings that I worried I might be

Around the same time, a friend of mine, Gemma, had a baby. During her pregnancy we'd exchanged emails about breastfeeding and I'd tried my best to give her helpful information. I first met Gemma's new baby when he was five weeks old and she informed me that she 'needed to talk boobs'. When we sat down to chat she told me how she had endured the most horrendous, painful thrush. She was now having to use nipple shields and was experiencing all kinds of anxieties about how that would affect their future success at breastfeeding. We had a chat and I did my best to make her feel better.

'You told me it gets easier after a few months and you should try your best to hang in there for six weeks if you can. It's been my mantra, it's kept me going when I desperately wanted to quit,' Gemma said.

It wasn't necessarily what I wanted to hear. I was glad I'd helped to keep her strong, but I felt I'd caused her to put up with pain and discomfort. Fortunately, she'd spoken to health professionals about the thrush and not just soldiered on through the pain. But I started to worry. At what point was my 'help' helpful? Could it be harmful? I realised I had to be very cautious about what I said and to whom. I worried I had overstepped the mark. I had a lot to learn.

One day, I spoke to the lady who now ran the breastfeeding group about what more I could do. She suggested trying peer supporter training and pointed me in the direction of a suitable course. You have to complete a module over the space of about two months in order to obtain your qualification, at which point you're basically a well-informed mum who can signpost other mothers to the right information and support

My module arrived and I looked through it. It didn't look too hard so I thought I would work on it when I had a moment. Suddenly, I found, with a month to spare, that I had barely done a thing! What with visiting Mum and looking after the kids, time had passed without me realising.

Fortunately, they gave me an extension and I finally finished it by working when I was putting Mae to bed; typing out my answers with the laptop on my knees while she fed. Over the years, I had learnt a lot of the *theory* of breastfeeding by trawling the internet, but I had a lot to learn about support. Completing the course I learned to think about what I said; how it might impact another mother. I learned to listen, reflect and really think about what help another mum might actually need. I wasn't advising mums about what they ought to be doing; I was a source of experience and support that they could choose to use or ignore.

It's always nice to get a certificate for something. Wearing my special volunteer T-shirt and chatting to mums at group was so rewarding that it quickly became the highlight of my week. I was 'doing my bit'.

Becoming a peer supporter caused me to reflect on my own experience. I could see now that a little help with positioning and attachment early on with Fin would have helped so much. Perhaps, even more importantly, more time spent chatting to other breastfeeding mums about what was normal would have helped me to stop beating myself up all the time.

The support that mums are able to give each other is just wonderful. Sometimes, as a peer supporter, you look at a room of mothers at different stages of their journey. Often, all they seem to be doing is swapping stories. But there's so much support in those interactions. The friendships made in these vulnerable times where you hold each other up are made of solid stuff. A community built from mutual support is a wonderful thing to be a part of. With the decline of the extended family, sometimes strangers take that place.

Now and then, I would see a woman come to our group looking haunted from her experiences but after some tea, cake and a chat, she would leave looking like a burden had been eased. I was so proud to play a small part in that. Even if women only came for a rant about what they had to face, just to get it off their chest, I knew how much it helped. We would all sit there, swap experiences, and relate to one another based on the struggles we faced in a society that didn't seem to understand our chosen mode of feeding.

As I look back on my experience, I can see that all too many health professionals, people paid to care for me, were misinformed or thoughtless (although there were also plenty who were wonderful). Even people with my best interests at heart would wound me with thoughtless comments and suggestions. But, whilst I had often felt like a breastfeeding island, it turned out that there were others out there, people who could say 'me too'. I wanted to help turn the tide, to make the world a kinder, better informed place.

When Mae was eight months old I decided to return to work. I was reluctant, having had a whole year with Fin, but I felt it was important to be back at the beginning of the school year if possible. Hesitantly, I started to make preparations.

In all honesty, I had been considering giving up work altogether. I couldn't see how I could possibly balance the stresses of full-time teaching with being a present parent to my two children (although I know plenty of people manage it). But my school gave me a great offer of a job-share that I couldn't refuse. It took the pressure off worrying about how to balance work and childcare and I hoped carrying on working would provide me with a little escapism, independence, and money.

I hadn't expressed milk at all for Mae up to this point; I hadn't needed to leave her. Now, I started to build up a stash in the freezer again but it was painfully slow; I would get half an ounce for a half hour pumping session. I knew it didn't mean that I had no milk, just that Mae was getting it, not the breast pump. It was going to take weeks to save up enough, meaning hours and hours of expressing in the lead up to my return to work.

I wondered how I was going to express at work. If I used my manual pump, would I have enough time to express during a break-time at school? I also worried about pupils hearing the clicking noise through the door and being curious as to what was going on.

I started to investigate electric breast pumps, but I didn't know where to start and they were quite expensive. Fortunately, Laura had one. She and Richard had their first son six months after Mae was born and Laura had expressed a lot for him in the early days. Just as I needed an electric pump she stopped using hers so she offered me an extended loan.

With the new pump I still didn't express a large quantity of milk, but at least it was quicker, didn't hurt my hand, and allowed me to multitask a little. I froze all the milk I was expressing before I went back to work in breast milk storage bags. I'd been given a good tip to freeze them on their side so that the milk is thinly spread across the bag. Then when you need the milk you can very quickly defrost it in some warm water. It meant I didn't have to get loads out of the freezer and risk it going bad; Angela could get it out as she needed it.

My boss was great. She offered me her office to express at work since it could be locked. She also arranged blinds to be put up over the glass in the doors. It was still weird having my chest bare on school premises, but at least I was secure. I kept my milk in a small cool bag in the staff fridge and nobody needed to be any the wiser of its contents.

When I got home the pot of breast milk would go straight in the fridge or freezer, ready to be decanted into a sippy cup the next day. Of course, Mae would no sooner take a bottle than her brother had, but this time it didn't particularly matter. I must say, I have the utmost respect for Angela handling my breast milk without so much as raising an eyebrow. I'm sure others might be squeamish.

I fell into a work routine quickly enough. Initially, I expressed at break-time and lunch. But break-time is short and I also needed time to photocopy sheets, go to the toilet and eat. I quickly dropped that session and only expressed at lunch, and still found it was sufficient to get enough milk for the next day. Expressing gave me a precious fifteen minutes in my day where I could simply sit and read or play with my phone. In such a hectic life, this was a lovely moment of peace.

Working two and a half days a week was much easier than full-time. I didn't feel so intensely that I was missing out. Sometimes, I struggled with the balance between work and childcare and I never got a rest from both. People don't always realise that both roles are intense and just because you don't work full-time in a paid role doesn't mean you aren't exhausted. The times when I used to get a respite from looking after two children, when Fin was in nursery, were now timed for when I was at work so that Angela had less to worry about. It was fair enough, but I was burning out.

I felt that if I complained then I would seem ungrateful. After all, I'd chosen to work and it wasn't as if I worked a lot. It was hard to admit that I needed space. Other people were sacrificing their time to enable me to work; I couldn't very well ask for more time so that I could sleep, read or sit alone for a while. I'd already been given enough. I felt like it was my duty to be on constant childcare duty when I was at home.

On top of this, I left work every day when the bell rang so that I could spend time with my children. Teachers do a great deal of work outside of the classroom and I had to take all that home with me. So, four nights a week, after the kids were in bed, I would get my books out for an hour, two hours, sometimes three when my brain was gooey and my eyes needed matchsticks. Now, I don't know about everybody else, but when the day's jobs are done I just want to get some brain space; some time to sit and vegetate. Sometimes, I like to sew or knit or read. But, the very last thing I want to do is to engage my brain and start working.

It's hard to cope with this kind of routine long term. But it was the choice I made. I could have stayed at work till six every night and seen the kids just long enough to kiss them goodnight. Or, I could have stayed at home and not worked. I chose the middle ground, which is perhaps harder than people realise.

When Mae was one I decided she no longer needed expressed milk. I wasn't keen on expressing anyway and could use the time productively at work. So, I decided she would have cow's milk on the days I wasn't there. She didn't even seem to notice the change; by this point she was only feeding in the mornings or when she needed a sleep anyway, so it wasn't a big deal.

Mae wasn't good with sleep but then, as I had come to realise, not many babies are. The prevailing idea that babies should sleep by whatever age makes me so cross. If we accept that they don't and ensure we have survival mechanisms it's so much easier to deal with than trying to fix a problem that isn't there.

As a small baby Mae had generally been a better sleeper than Fin; she maybe woke three times a night where he woke four or five. I could generally get her to sleep in her cot and hadn't needed to employ a dummy. On the other hand, Fin slept through the night reliably at ten months. Ten months came and went and Mae still woke at night.

It's all well and good having disrupted sleep when you have some hope of organising your day to include a nap, but this was out of the question now. I had to power on, working or running after a toddler, often wondering how I was still standing. I tried to stop worrying about when she would sleep through the night, knowing that it would happen eventually.

Still, I kept working on getting Mae to sleep better. She definitely needed a good meal in her to help her to sleep but there didn't seem to be much else I could do. But, without doing very much at all, she slowly started to settle for longer. We had good nights and bad nights but, generally, on a bad night she would come and snuggle in our bed and the worst thing was trying to sleep with her sleeping horizontally between Stuart and I.

When Mae was one she took a serious dislike to her cot. She would desperately try to get out (and looked scarily like she could be capable of doing it). Also, I was struggling to put her gently down in the cot when she was asleep. As your child gets older you have to lower the base of the cot. Initially, when they're tiny, you can have it high to save your back. But, then, as they become more mobile you lower the base to keep them from toppling out. I'm not really tall enough to lower a sleeping one-year-old down almost to floor level so the last few inches would often be a fumble that would wake her. Anyway, we resorted to often getting her out of the cot, putting her mattress on the floor and then lying with her and settling her there. This became such a habit that it seemed silly to still be bothering with the cot. It was time for a big girl bed.

I was concerned that it was 'too early', but Mae had been sleeping without bars for a while, so really there was no change. Also, with respect to her climbing ability, this was safer. Everything she could get access to upstairs was safe and there was a stair gate at the top of the stairs. Putting Mae in a toddler bed was great. She could get up in the night and come to us, meaning that I didn't need to go and get her any more. In the evening, I would lie comfortably with her in her toddler bed (one of the advantages of being short), while I fed her, and then sneak off once she was asleep.

Fin's sleeplessness had seemed agonising and everlasting. But Mae's waking, whilst not as frequent, went on and on. She would wake for feeds that I was convinced she didn't need (having had milk and food all day). I tried giving her lots of daytime feeds to make her less likely to want them at night, but it didn't seem to help.

It was time to try to night wean Mae. She seemed to only want milk when I was around so I put Stuart in charge. When Mae woke in the night, he would go and soothe her. Or, if she made it to our bed before he got up, I would leave and sleep in the spare room. Stuart would snuggle Mae up and she would go right off to sleep with no milk. Before too long she was going long stretches at night and, when she did wake, a cuddle from either one of us would do the trick as the link between me and night-time milk had been broken.

Before I knew it, Mae had dropped all but the bedtime feed. For the most part, it was a lovely time of day. I would snuggle up with her in her bed and feed her while messing around on my iPad. I got to have a lie down in a dimly lit room and switch off. Even if I had to go and do schoolwork afterwards, at least I had that moment of calm.

However, as Mae grew, she became very talented at 'gymnurstics', much as her brother before her. She would fidget, climb on me, turn so that her body was in the opposite direction to mine or clamber over me from one side to the other. All of this would take place with her latched on. Not only was my nipple being dragged every which way, but it was seriously annoying being a climbing frame.

I also began to find that, sometimes, feeding made me cringe again, just like the first time around. Interestingly, mammalian mothers can get aggressive around weaning time[1] and I wonder whether the negative feelings that I felt, meaning that I had to grit my teeth to feed without losing my temper, suggested that our time was coming to an end. But then I wonder whether it was triggered by the fact that I fed so little, I wasn't used to it any more. I was definitely 'touched out' that's for sure. I was tired of having the children touching me all the time.

I had mixed feeling about feeding by this point, just as with Fin. Breastfeeding was amazing, but sometimes I didn't want to do it. I had wanted to hit the two year mark this time. But then, what is a number? Did it matter if it was two years, or a bit before?

One night, I decided I wouldn't breastfeed Mae; I'd had enough. She was nineteen months old and cheekier than you would believe. We went through the normal routine: bath, pyjamas, story and then into bed. Mae sat in the middle of that big toddler bed looking at me with her saucer eyes as I sat cross-legged on the floor next to her.

'Lie down then,' I said, sweetly. Mae vigorously shook her head, curly hair swinging about her face. 'Go on, lie down,' I repeated. She did, whilst still looking at me, trying to communicate through her eyes what she wanted. Then, she grinned at me and patted the bed next to her. I laughed and hopped into bed and fed her.

I told this story to Stuart. The next night he asked me if I wanted to stop feeding and offered to put Mae to bed. Reluctantly, I said yes. I realised that, for me, the time had come, provided that she wasn't too heartbroken. So, Stuart got our little girl into her pyjamas and took her off to bed.

Stuart sent Mae in to say goodnight. She kissed Fin and then kissed me, fixed me with that steely stare, plonked herself down in my lap and refused to shift. When Stuart came to get her she resisted but, as soon as she was out of my sight, she happily went to have her book and go to sleep. A similar pattern emerged for the next few nights. She would try to get me to come with her, but once I said no she would go peacefully.

Our whole routine changed as we got the opportunity to bond at night-time with the 'other child'. I got to do the bedtime stories with Fin that I had missed for almost two years. After all, I did have two children, and my eldest had very much been pushed towards Daddy so that I could feed his sister. Now I got to spend more time with my firstborn. We would snuggle up in bed together to read his books. It was bliss.

Stuart got into the habit of giving Mae books to look at as she fell asleep. I liked that. I've fallen asleep reading many, many times in my life and I couldn't object to such a peaceful drift into sleep. No tears, no 'crying it out', just a happy, grown-up girl who didn't have her milk any more.

It was a few days before it really hit me. I was at the fridge pouring some cow's milk into a beaker for the little terror standing in front of me. Mae could walk and talk and be mischievous and she now only had cow's milk, milk from another species. I had often wondered how long I would feed her for. Here was my answer, nineteen months and twenty-two days; my 'personal best'.

31

THIRD TIME LUCKY

It seemed unlikely I would feed another baby. But, as Mae reached school age and we still hadn't got rid of the loft full of baby clothes, we realised we probably weren't quite done with this…and here I am with my third baby lying across my arms, snoring while I type.

Pregnancy was rough. When the constant nausea of the first trimester abated, my hands and feet erupted in eczema that I clawed until it bled. Then, my skin repeatedly peeled off, leaving it cracked and scarred. I had sinusitis about five times, which just seemed unfair. PGP reared its head again about halfway through the pregnancy making it virtually impossible to move and so helping me to pile on three stone. I felt the difference with this being a third pregnancy, compared to a first, and with me being thirty-two years old, compared to twenty-six.

We decided not to find out the sex of the baby. We had no practical need since we'd kept clothes and toys from Fin and Mae. The baby would be starting out in our bedroom so there was no need to fret over whose room it would share, we could figure out that sort of thing once it was here. We thought it would be fun to find out on the day, although it drove everybody to distraction guessing.

I wanted another home birth, since Mae's birth had been so amazing, but it didn't work out thanks to my waters breaking early. I was told I had twenty-four hours to give birth at home before I would need to go to hospital for antibiotics due to the infection risk to us both.[1] The baby took its sweet time so we ended up back in the hospital where Fin was born. That was fine, though; I knew what I wanted and I was strong enough to stand up for myself.

The consultant-led unit now has a birthing pool, so with an IV in my arm for the antibiotics I laboured for hours in the water. The midwife suggested I shift position and I instantly lost all of my focus. The pain became too much and I panicked that I might end up suffering as much as I did during my labour with Fin.

'Please, I need an epidural,' I begged.

'You're doing beautifully, perhaps try a different position.'

'No…I've had enough. I can't take any more,' I cried through tears of panic. The midwife agreed to get me an epidural and got me out of the pool. She walked me to the room next door to where Fin was born. I was disappointed, but empowered that I had made the choice I needed to make. I had nothing to prove. If I needed respite then that was fine.

At the door I felt that all-too-familiar pressure. I rushed to grip the bed, hearing the midwife reassure me, 'Don't worry; it looks as though baby's coming right here!'

Moments later, I passed the tiniest baby through my legs,

just six and a half pounds as it turned out. I clambered on to the bed and laid the baby on my chest where it nuzzled in and started to snore. I remembered suddenly that I had no idea what sex this baby was. I lifted it and peeked

'Oh, it's a girl!' I cried in surprise.

'Oh wow! Another girl,' Stuart said. We had a boy name and a girl name ready; now we knew which we would be using. I looked at the midwife.

'This is Zoe,' I said.

Some hours later, my mum brought Zoe's siblings to meet her. First to peek round my curtain was six-year-old Fin, frowning. He'd been anxiously awaiting the news of Zoe's arrival at school; it hadn't crossed my mind to get the message to him that she had been born. Four-year-old Mae, on the other hand, had found out straight away from my mum and had been bouncing up and down shouting, 'I've got a sister,' at the top of her lungs.

I held my arms open and Fin ran to me for a hug, needing to know his mum was OK more than he needed to see his new sister. Mae, with a furtive grin, crept over to the baby leading my mum by the hand. Mae's face bloomed with delight as she saw the baby she had been waiting so long to meet.

Watching my older children holding their tiny baby sister was one of the most special moments of my life. They were in love with her from that first moment. Even Fin, who had been unconvinced as a toddler at the arrival of Mae, was obviously besotted with tiny Zoe.

Breastfeeding wasn't all plain sailing. I hoped to start out with a breast crawl but, yet again, it didn't happen. Zoe was just too tired and I wanted to speed up the delivery of the placenta. In the end I hurried her up and got her feeding myself.

Even in that first feed I could see that latching wasn't easy for Zoe. She struggled to get suction and clicked and slurped as she lost grip on my nipple. Within hours I was starting to get sore. I texted a friend from breastfeeding group who arrived at my house moments after I got home. She confirmed my suspicions that Zoe probably had a tongue-tie.

We all have a degree of tongue-tie, that flap of skin that anchors your tongue to your mouth, but for some babies it's so tight that they can't properly manoeuvre their tongues.[2(pp428-429)] Zoe's was so restricted that the tip was pulled in; her tongue was heart-shaped. Fortunately, it was something with which I was familiar since my nephew had been born with the same issue.

Rather than being referred for an official diagnosis I decided to see how things went. On occasion, the effects of a tongue-tie can sort themselves out and I felt I could cope for the time being. In the meantime, I was meticulous about latching Zoe on perfectly so that I could minimise any damage to my nipples.

Zoe regained her birth weight very quickly; her tongue-tie has never compromised her ability to put on weight, otherwise I would have had it divided. At such a young age this procedure is just a quick snip without even any anaesthetic; it wouldn't have been a big deal.[2(p430)] However, after a few initial days of soreness we managed to get a sufficiently good latch that her tongue-tie wasn't an issue, except the slurping noises she persisted in making, particularly when I was feeding around men.

Having experienced tongue-tie and being sufficiently knowledgeable and supported to know what it was, I wonder if Fin had one too. Perhaps, that's why I was in pain in those early days, and the reason his weight was often an issue. I will never know for sure but I have my suspicions. If only I'd had the same level of support back then that I have now, I would have been able to deal with it as ably as I did this time.

One day, I went to a baby massage class. I was in a great, confident mood. I'd been living in a rosy bubble since Zoe's birth. She, however, was cantankerous and wouldn't stop crying; I arrived flustered because I was late. Added to that, I was annoyed because I wasn't welcomed; I just had an empty spot gestured to me.

I sat, dumped my stuff, and latched Zoe on, assuming a feed would sort her out. As I struggled to breastfeed this ball of fury I noticed people glancing at me. I felt paranoid that I was being judged for this baby that clearly didn't want to feed, even though, in hindsight, I doubt that was what anyone was thinking. I looked for the solidarity of another breastfeeding mum giving me that look of 'we've all been there'. I didn't see it.

Zoe calmed and I tried joining in with the class and massaging her a little. I glanced around, seeing two or three mums bottle-feeding their babies, but nobody breastfeeding.

Zoe started fussing again and, yet again, I was the only lady with her breasts out (and with the flailing baby there can't have been anyone who didn't catch a glimpse). The lady running the group said, to the group in general, 'If you need to feed your babies you can go over there,' pointing to a set of chairs at one end of the room where two women were bottle-feeding. I felt the comment was directed at me so I got up and joined them.

Zoe kept crying and I felt increasingly uncomfortable, despite the sympathetic smiles of the bottle-feeding mums sat with me. I suddenly became very self-aware, almost like an out-of-body experience. I realised I was shaking; I was feeling the same anxiety that I used to feel with Fin all those years ago, in those groups with everyone discussing how many ounces their babies drank and how long they slept. I hadn't felt like that in years.

I grabbed my stuff and ran. Sitting in the car with tears streaming down my face, I realised that, in the village of wonderful support that I now inhabited, I had forgotten how alien it can feel to be the only woman breastfeeding; the only woman baring her chest and feeling judged for doing so (even if, on this particular day, it was all in my head). I was so used to only hanging out with mum friends I already knew and feeling totally comfortable with breastfeeding around them, especially since most were people from breastfeeding group, I'd forgotten how unusual it was to breastfeed in the world outside my bubble. Having breastfed, on and off, for seven years I could still feel uncomfortable breastfeeding in public. So much has changed, and yet also so little.

Stuart and I feel done with having babies and are enjoying every moment of this last time. It might be chaos, and it's far from perfect, but it's wonderful nonetheless.

Breastfeeding will forever hold a sacred place in my heart and will always be one of the most cherished parts of my children's infancy. Those early days with Fin might have been tough, but they taught me so much about who I am and about the journeys that other women have to take. Motherhood isn't easy, and I think we tend to forget how lonely and arduous it can be.

I have learnt so much about breastfeeding, from history, to politics, to science and from my own personal experience. I never, for a moment, expected it to be so interesting and fulfilling. Who knew that breastfeeding was anything more than just feeding a baby?

There's so much that needs addressing. In a society that talks an awful lot about feminism, why are women still being marginalised and made to feel guilty for doing something central to our survival as a species and something that is fundamentally female? Why are women hiding breastfeeding as if it's a shameful thing? Why are mothers being pitted against mothers when the fight is surely nothing to do with competition, but rather about the right to feed your child in the way that you wish? Why do women who want to breastfeed not find the support in their communities to do so? I still hope that one day breastfeeding becomes a boring topic of conversation because it's so unexceptional and familiar. I hope we look back and marvel at how topsy-turvy infant feeding had become.

We need to fill our communities with information,

experience and compassion so that women don't suffer when there's no need; so they are prepared and know where to turn. We need to be honest about what's normal for mothers and babies and remove this strange ideal that serves only to cause guilt and strain. We should feel able to talk openly about our stories, to reach out for help or be a source of experience to somebody else.

I was fortunate to see what good support looked like when I had Mae. It healed my wounds. Whilst I wish life had been easier in the early days with Fin, I wouldn't have been driven to care so much about breastfeeding so, in part, I can be grateful for that experience. Now, I get to help other mothers as a peer supporter and 'do my bit' to make breastfeeding easier.

Our little Zoe has taught me that breastfeeding with a support network can be wonderful, even with difficulties. She's taught me just how important my 'village' is. The struggles I had when my family and friends knew little about breastfeeding no longer exist now my peers are knowledgeable and supportive. But there's still a lot of change needed in our society for mothers, and I mean *all* mothers, to feel supported and empowered in motherhood.

Breastfeeding, of course, is highly personal. For me, it made me who I am; not only the mother that I am, but the person I am. I'm more selfless, more empathetic, and more driven. I recognise the strength in motherhood, in womanhood in general, and the importance of equality and compassion more than I ever did before.

Breastfeeding shaped our family. It changed my life, *our* lives, and I am so very grateful

REFERENCES

Chapter 1: Breastfeeding and Me

None

Chapter 2: Mammals and Mammaries

1. Phillips MJ, Bennett TH, Lee MSY (2009) Molecules, morphology, and ecology indicate a recent, amphibious ancestry for echidnas. *Proc Natl Acad Sci USA*.106:17089–1709.
2. Schiebinger L. Why Mammals are Called Mammals: Gender Politics in Eighteenth-Century Natural History. *Am Hist Rev*. 1993, Apr;98(2):382–411.
3. Attenborough D. *The Life of Mammals*. London: BBC Books; 2002.
4. Purves WK, Sadava D, Orians, GH, Heller HC. *Life: The Science of Biology*. 6th ed. Sunderland, MA: Sinauer Associates; 2001. p593.
5. Richardson K. *Australia's Amazing Kangaroos: Their Conservation, Unique Biology and Coexistence with Humans*. Collingwood, Australia: Csiro; 2012. p41.
6. Johnson SA, editor. *Bats*. Adaptation of Masuda M. Kōmori (Jacobsen WM, Trans.). Lerner Publications Company; 1985. p27-32.

7. Boness DJ, Clapham PJ, Mesnick SL. Life histories and reproductive strategies. In: Hoelzel AR, editor. *Marine Mammal Biology*. Oxford: Blackwell Sciences Ltd; 2002. p278-324.
8. Oftedal OT. Use of maternal reserves as a lactation strategy in large mammals. *Proc Nutr Soc.* 2000, Feb;59(1):99-106.
9. Lockyer C. Review of Baleen Whale (Mysticeti Reproduction and Implications for Management. In: Report - International Whaling Commission. 1984, Jan;6:27:50.
10. Oftedal OT. Lactation in Whales and Dolphins: Evidence of Divergence Between Baleen- and Toothed Species. *J Mammary Gland Biol Neoplasia.* 1997, Jul;2(3):205-230.
11. Cowardine M. *Whales, Dolphins and Porpoises.* London: Dorling Kindersley; 1995. p11.
12. Johnson G, Frantzis A, Johnson C, Alexiadou V, Ridgway S. Evidence that sperm whale (Physeter macrocephalus) calves suckle through their mouth. *Mar. Mamm. Sci.* 2010, Oct;26(4):990-996.
13. Sakalidis VS, Geddes DT. Suck-Swallow-Breathe Dynamics in Breastfed Infants. *J Hum Lact.* 2016, May;32(2):201-211.
14. Hinde K, Milligan LA. Primate Milk: Proximate Mechanisms and Ultimate Perspectives. *Evolutionary Anthropology.* 2011, Jan-Feb;20(1):9-23.
15. Sherman PW, Braude S, Jarvis JUM. Litter sizes and mammary numbers of naked mole-rats: breaking the one-half rule. *J Mammal.* 1999, Aug;80(3):720-733.
16. Velanovich V. Ectopic breast tissue, supernumerary breasts and supernumerary nipples. *South Med J.* 1995, Sep;88(9):903-6.
17. Kunz H, Hosen DJ. Male lactation: why, why not and is it care? *Trends Ecol Evol.* 2009, Feb;24(2):80-85.
18.
19. McClellen HL, Miller SJ, Hartman PE. Evolution of lactation: nutrition v protection with special reference to five mammalian species. *Nutr Res Rev.* 2008, Dec;21(2):97-116.

Chapter 3: Life Before Babies

1. Wiessinger D, West D, Pitman T, *The Womanly Art of Breastfeeding.* 8th ed. London: Pinter and Martin; 2010. p14.

Chapter 4: Milk

1. Rapley G, Murkett T. *Baby-led Breastfeeding.* London: Vermilion; 2012.
2. Evans, K. *The Food of Love.* Brighton: Myriad Editions; 2009.
3. Harman T, Wakeford A. *The Microbiome Effect.* London: Pinter and Martin; 2016.
4. Mueller NT, Bakacs E, Combellick J, Grigoryan Z, Dominguez-Bello MG. The infant microbiome development: mom matters. *Trends Mol Med.* 2015, Feb;21(2):109-117.
5. Cabrera-Rubio R, Collado MC, Laitinen K, Salminen S, Isolauri E, and Mira A. The human milk microbiome changes over lactation and is shaped by maternal weight and mode of delivery. *Am J Clin Nutr.* 2012, Sep;96(3)544-551.
6. Sears W, Sears M. *The Baby Book.* 2nd ed. London: Thorsons; 2005. p117-122.
7. Daly SJ, Di Rosso A, Owens RA, Hartmann PE. Degree of breast emptying explains changes in the fat content, but not fatty acid composition, of human milk. *Exp Physiol.* 1993, Nov;78(6):741-55.
8. Cubero J, Valero V, Sanchez J, Rivero M, Parvez H, Rodriguez AB, Barriga C. The circadian rhythm of tryptophan in breast milk affects the rhythms of 6-sulfatoxymelatonin and sleep in newborn. *Nuero Endocrinol Lett,* 2005, Dec;26(6):657-61.
9. Rapley G, Murkett T. *Baby-led Breastfeeding.* London: Vermilion; 2012. p29-30.
10. Fujita M, Roth E, Lo YJ, Hurst C, Vollner J, Kendell A. In poor families, mothers' milk is richer for daughters than sons: A test of Trivers-Willard hypothesis in agropastoral settlements in Northern Kenya. *Am J Phys Anthropol.* 2012, Sep;149:52-59.
11. Khan S, Hepworth AR, Prime DK, Lai CT, Trengove NJ. Hartmann PE. Variation in fat, lactose, and protein composition in breast milk over 24 hours: associations with infant feeding patterns. *J Hum Lact.* 2013, Feb;29(1):81-89.

12. Ludington-How SM, Lewis T, Cong X, Anderson L. Breast-Infant Temperature with Twins during Shared Kangaroo Care. *J Obstet Gynecol Neonatal Nurs.* 2006;35(2):223-231.
13. Hill PD, Chatterton Jr RT, Aldag J.C. Serum Prolactin in Breast-feeding: State of the Science. *Biol Res Nurs* 1999, Jul;1(1):65-75.
14. Evans, K. *The Food of Love.* Brighton: Myriad Editions; 2009. p10.
15. Uvnas Moberg, K. *The Oxytocin Factor.* London: Pinter and Martin; 2011. p65.
16. Rapley G, Murkett T. *Baby-led Breastfeeding.* London: Vermilion; 2012. p24.
17. Wiessinger D, West D, Pitman T, *The Womanly Art of Breastfeeding.* 8th ed. London: Pinter and Martin; 2010. p43.

Chapter 5: Love Story

1. Ebisch IMW, Thomas CMG, Peters WHM, Braat DDM, Steegers-Theunissen RPM. The importance of folate, zinc and antioxidants in the pathogenesis and prevention of subfertility. *Hum Reprod Update.* 2007, Mar-Apr;13(2):163-74.
2. MRC Vitamin Study Research Group. Prevention of neural tube defects: Results of the Medical Research Council Vitamin Study. *Lancet.* 1991, Jul;338(8760):131.137.
3. Sedgwick Harvey MA, McRorie MM, Smith DW. Suggested limits to the use of hot tub and sauna by pregnant women. *Can Med Assoc J.* 1981, Jul, 1;125(1):50-53.

Chapter 6: The History of Breastfeeding

1. Palmer G. *The Politics of Breastfeeding.* London: Pinter and Martin; 2009.
2. Grayson J. *Unlatched: The Evolution of Breastfeeding and the Making of a Controversy.* New York: Harper Collins; 2016.

3. Konner M, Worthman C. Nursing Frequency, Gonadal Function and Birth Spacing among !Kung Hinter Gatherers. *Science*. 1980, Feb;207(4432):788-91.

4. Stevens EE, Patrick TE, Picklor R. A History of Infant Feeding. *J Perinat Educ*. 2009, Spring;18(2):32-39.

5. Exodus 2:8, Holy Bible.

6. Thorvaldsen G. Was there a European breastfeeding pattern? *Hist Fam*. 2008, Sep;13(3):283-295.

7. Salmon M. The cultural significance of breastfeeding and infant care in early modern England and America. *J Soc Hist*. 1994, Winter;28(2):247-269.

8. Schiebinger L. Why Mammals are Called Mammals: Gender Politics in Eighteenth-Century Natural History. *Am Hist Rev*. 1993, Apr;98(2):382–411.

9. Rousseau, J.J. *Emile*. 1763 [reprint] London: J.M. Dent and Sons; 1992. p13.

10. Qur'an 31:14. Madina, King Fahd Hold Qur'an Printing Complex; 1410 H.

11. Yashmin S. Islamic and Cultural Practices in Breastfeeding. [Internet]. *Leader Today*; October 1 2015. Available from: http://leadertoday.breastfeedingtoday-llli.org/islamic-and-cultural-practices-in-breastfeeding/ [cited June 12 2018].

12. Parkes P. Milk kinship in Islam. Substance, structure, history. *Social Anthropology*. 2005, Jan, 19;13(3) 307-329.

13. Valenze D. *Milk: A Local and Global History*. New Haven and London: Yale University Press; 2011. p159.

14. Svanborg C, Agerstam H, Aronson A, Bjerkvig R, Duringer C, Fischer W, Gustafsson L, Hallgren O, Leijonhuvud I, Linse S, Mossberg AK, Nilsson H, Pettersson J, Svensson, M. HAMLET kills tumor cells by an apoptosis-like mechanism-Cellular, molecular, and therapeutic aspects. *Adv Cancer Res*. 2003;88:1–29.

15. Takeuchi M. Breastfeeding in Japan: historical perspectives and current attitudes and practices. *Jpn Hosp* 1992, Jul;11:79–92.

16. Brown A. *Breastfeeding Uncovered: Who Really Decides How We Feed Our Babies*. London: Pinter and Martin; 2016. p159-168.

Chapter 7: Waiting for Baby

1. Rapley G, Murkett T. *Baby-led Breastfeeding.* London: Vermilion; 2012. p15.
2. Cooke K. *The Rough Guide to Pregnancy and Birth.* London: Rough Guides; 2010. p137.

Chapter 8: The World we Feed in

1. Stevens EE, Patrick TE, Pickler R. A History of Infant Feeding. *J Perinat Educ.* 2009, Spring;18(2):32-39
2. Grayson J. *Unlatched: The Evolution of Breastfeeding and the Making of a Controversy.* New York: Harper Collins; 2016.
3. Palmer G. *The Politics of Breastfeeding.* London: Pinter and Martin; 2009.
4. Radbill S. Infant feeding through the ages. *Clin Pediatr (Phila).* 1981, Oct;20(10), 613–21.
5. Brown A. *Breastfeeding Uncovered: Who Really Decides How We Fed Our Babies.* London: Pinter and Martin; 2016.
6. Sears W, Sears M. *The Baby Book.* 2nd ed. London: Thorsons; 2005.
7. NHS Choices. How to make up baby formula. [Internet] Available from: https://www.nhs.uk/conditions/pregnancy-and-baby/making-up-infant-formula/ [cited 18 May 2018].
8. Newman J, Pitman T. *The Ultimate Breastfeeding Book of Answers.* Rosevikke, California: Prima Publishing; 2000. p26-27.
9. Baby Milk Action [internet]. Available from www.babymilkaction.org [cited 30th March 2017].
10. World Health Organization (WHO), Unicef. The International Code of Marketing of Breast-milk Substitutes. Geneva: WHO; 1981.
11. World Health Organization (WHO). Marketing of breast-milk substitutes: national implementation of the international code. Status report 2016. Geneva, WHO; 2016.

12. The Infant Formula and Follow-on Formula (England) Regulations 2007. No 3521.

13. World Health Organization (WHO) Information concerning the use and marketing of follow up formula. [Internet] Geneva, WHO; 2013. Available from: http://www.who.int/nutrition/topics/WHO_brief_fufandcode_post_17July.pdf [cited May 10 2017]

14. La Leche League International. A brief history of La Leche League International. [Internet]. Available from: https://www.llli.org/about/history/ [cited June 15 2018].

15. Association of Breastfeeding Mothers (ABM). Training. [Internet] Available from: https://abm.me.uk/breastfeeding-training/ [cited June 14 2018].

16. The Breastfeeding Network. Peer Supporter Projects. [Internet] Available from: https://www.breastfeedingnetwork.org.uk/get-involved/train-to-be-a-registered-volunteer/peer-support-programmes/ [cited June 13 2018].

17. Scott JA, Mostyn T. Women's experiences of breastfeeding in a bottlefeeding culture. *J Hum Lact*. 2003 Aug;19(3):270-7.

18. Equality Act; 2010 (c. 15).

19. Nadvornak, D. Breastfeeding Bill Passes Idaho Legislature. [internet] Spokane public radio; 2018. Available from: http://spokanepublicradio.org/post/breastfeeding-bill-passes-idaho-legislature [cited Jun 16 2018].

20. Murphy E. Risk, Responsibilty, and Rhetoric in Infant Feeding. *J Contemp Ethnogr*, 2000, Jun;29(3):291-325.

21. Marshall JL, Godfrey M, Renfrew MJ. Being a 'good mother': Managing breastfeeding and merging identities. *Soc Sci Med*. 2007, Nov;65(10):2147-59.

22. Martin CR, Redshaw M. Editorial. Is breast always best? Balancing benefits and Choice. *J Reprod Infant Psychol*. 2011;29(2):113-114.

Chapter 9: Preparations

1. Rapley G, Murkett T. *Baby-led Breastfeeding*. London: Vermilion; 2012.
2. World Health Organization (WHO). Global strategy for infant and young child feeding. Geneva, WHO; 2003:p8.

Chapter 10: Having Babies

1. Gupta JK, Nikodem VC. Women's position during second stage of labour. *Cochrane Database Syst Rev*. 2000;(2):CD002006.
2. Sears W, Sears M. *The Baby Book*. 2nd ed. London: Thorsons; 2005. p25.
3. Barnett R. A horse named 'Twilight Sleep': the language of obstetric anaesthesia in 20th century Britain. *Int J Obstet Anesth*. 2005, Oct;14(4):310-5.
4. Leavitt JW. Birthing and Anesthesia: The Debate over Twilight Sleep. *Signs*. 1980;6(1);147–164.
5. *Mad Men*. The Fog. 2009; Series 3, Episode 5.
6. Palmer G. *The Politics of Breastfeeding*. London: Pinter and Martin; 2009.
7. Thomasson MA. Treber, J, 2008. From home to hospital: The evolution of childbirth in the United States, 1928-1940, *Explor Econ Hist*. 2008, Jan;45(1):76-99.
8. Brown A. *Breastfeeding Uncovered: Who Really Decides How We Feed Our Babies*. London: Pinter and Martin; 2016.
9. Johanson R, Newburn M, Macfarlane A. Has the medicalisation of birth gone too far. BMJ. 2002, Apr,13;324(7342):892-5.
10. NHS Digital. NHS Maternity Statistics 2016-2017. [Internet]. Health and Social Care Information Centre; 2017. Available from: https://files.digital.nhs.uk/pdf/l/1/hosp-epis-stat-mat-repo-2016-17.pdf [cited June 4 2018].
11. Uvnas Moberg, K. *The Oxytocin Factor*. London: Pinter and Martin; 2011. p69-70.

12. Ueda T, Yokoyama Y, Irahara M, Aono T. Influence of psychological stress on suckling-induced pulsatile oxytocin release. *Obstet Gynecol*. 1984, Aug;84(2):259-62.

13. Wiessinger D, West D, Pitman T, *The Womanly Art of Breastfeeding*. 8th ed. London: Pinter and Martin; 2010. p44.

14. Jiang H. Quian X, Carroli G, Garner P. Selective versus routine use of episiotomy for vaginal birth. *Cochrane Database Syst Rev*; 2017, Feb, 8;(2):CD000081.

15. Zanardo V, Svegliado G, Cavallin F, Giustardi A, Cosmi E, Litta P, Trevisanuto D. Elective Cesarean Delivery: Does It Have a Negative Effect on Breastfeeding. *Birth*. 2010, Dec;37(4):275-279.

16. Nissen E, Uvnäs-Moberg K, Svensson K, Stock S, Widström A, Winberg J. Different patterns of oxytocin, prolactin but not cortisol release during breastfeeding in women delivered by Caesarean section or by the vaginal route. *Early Hum Dev*. 1996, Jul;45(1-2):103-18.

17. Rowe-Murray HJ, Fisher JRW. Baby Friendly Hospital Practices: Cesarean Section is a Persistent Barrier to Early Initiation of Breastfeeding. *Birth*. 2002, Jun;29(2):124-31.

18. Jordan S, Emery S, Bradshaw C, Watkins A, Friswell W. The impact of intrapartum analgesia on infant feeding. *BJOG*. 2005, Jul;112(7):927-934.

19. Torvalden S, Roberts CL, Simpson JM, Thompson JF, Ellwood DA. Intrapartum epidural analgesia and breastfeeding: a prospective cohort study. *Int Breastfeed J* [Internet] 2006 [cited 10th June 2018];1:24. Available from doi: 10.1186/1746-4358-1-24.

20. Lieberman E, Lang JM, Cohen A, D'Agostino R Jr, Datta S, Frigoletto FD Jr. Association of epidural analgesa with caesarean delivery in nulliparas. *Obstet Gynecol*. 1996 Dec;88(6) 993-1000.

21. Rahm V, Hallgren A, Högberg H, Hurtig I, Odling V. Plasma oxytocin levels in women during labour with or without epidural analgesia: a prospective study. *Acta Obstet Gynecol Scand*. 2002, Nov;81(11):1033-9.

22. Crenshaw JT. Healthy Birth Practice #6: Keep Mother and Baby Together- It's Best for Mother, Baby and Breastfeeding. *J Perinat Educ*. 2014, Fall; 23(4):211-217.

Chapter 11: Birth

1. Gurgle.com. *Pregnancy: How to Enjoy It.* London: London: HarperCollins; 2009. p119.
2. Botelli SE, Locatelli A, Nespoli A. Early pushing in labour and midwifery practice: A prospective observational study in an Italian maternity hospital. *Midwifery.* 2013, Aug;29(8):871-875.
3. Steen M. *Pregnancy & Birth.* London: Dorling Kindersley; 2011. p112.

Chapter 12: How to Breastfeed

1. Rapley G, Murkett T. *Baby-led Breastfeeding.* London: Vermilion; 2012.
2. Wiessinger D, West D, Pitman T, *The Womanly Art of Breastfeeding.* 8th ed. London: Pinter and Martin; 2010.
3. Brown A. *Breastfeeding Uncovered: Who Really Decides How We Feed Our Babies.* London: Pinter and Martin; 2016. p78-80.
4. Niala C. Why African Babies Don't Cry: An African Perspective. [Internet]. The Natural Child Project: blog. Available from: http://www.naturalchild.org/guest/claire_niala.html [cited 13 December 2017].

Chapter 13: Crazy

1. Peck S. 2014. Bounty Mutiny victory for Mumsnet: sales reps should be banned from NHS maternity wards. *The Telegraph* [Internet] www.telegraph.co.uk/women/mother-tongue/10970286/Bounty-Mutiny-victory-for-Mumsnet-sales-reps-should-be-banned-from-NHS-maternity-wards.html [cited 8 May 2017].

Chapter 14: Most People Breastfeed, Right?

1. World Health Organization (WHO). Global strategy for infant and young child feeding. Geneva, WHO; 2003.
2. McAndrew F, Thompson, J, Fellows L, Large A, Speed M, Renfrew MJ. Infant Feeding Survey 2010. The Health and Social Care information Centre; 2012.
3. Centers for Disease Control and Prevention (CDC). Breastfeeding Report Card: Progressing toward national breastfeeding goals. United States, 2016. Atlanta, GA: National Centre for Chronic Disease Prevention and Health Promotion, Division of Nutrition, Physical Activity and Obesity; 2016.
4. Brown A. *Breastfeeding Uncovered: Who Really Decides How We Feed Our Babies.* London: Pinter and Martin; 2016.
5. Unicef, World Health Organisation (WHO) Global Breastfeeding Scorecard, 2017. Tracking Progress for Breastfeeding Policies and Programmes. New York: Unicef, Geneva:WHO; 2017.
6. Rapley G, Murkett T. *Baby-led Breastfeeding.* London: Vermilion; 2012. p211-212.
7. Akre JE, Gribble KD, Minchin M. Milk sharing: from private practice to public pursuit. *Int Breastfeed J.* [Internet] 2011 [cited 3 Jun 2018]; 6(8). Available from doi 10.1186/1746-4358-6-8
8. Thorley V. Sharing Breastmilk: Wet Nursing, Cross-feeding, and Milk Donations. *Breastfeed Rev.* 2008, Mar;16(1):25-9.

Chapter 15: Blood, Sweat and Tears

1. Wiessinger D, West D, Pitman T, *The Womanly Art of Breastfeeding.* 8th ed. London: Pinter and Martin; 2010. p88.
2. Palmer G. *The Politics of Breastfeeding.* London: Pinter and Martin; 2009. p37 & p53.
3. Hunt C, Fogle, M. *The Bump Class.* London: Vermillion; 2016. p178.
4. Rapley G, Murkett T. *Baby-led Breastfeeding.* London: Vermilion; 2012. p38.

5. Jones, W. Analgesics (painkillers) and Breastfeeding. Paisley: The Breastfeeding Network;2004. Available from: https://www.breastfeedingnetwork.org.uk/wp-content/dibm/analgesics.pdf [cited 21st March 2016].

6. Buchanan P, Hands A, Jones W. Assessing the evidence: Cracked Nipples and Moist Wound Healing. Paisley: The Breastfeeding Network; Mar 2002. Available from https://www.breastfeedingnetwork.org.uk/wp-con-tent/pdfs/Cracked_Nipples_and_Moist_Wound_Healing_2002.pdf [cited Jan 2017].

7. World Health Organization (WHO). Global strategy for infant and young child feeding. Geneva, WHO; 2003.

Chapter 16: Trying Times

1. Hoddinott P, Kroll T, Raja A, Lee AJ. Seeing other women breastfeed: how vicarious experience relates to breastfeeding intention and behaviour. *Matern Child Nutr.* 2010, Apr, 6(2):134-46.

2. Wiessinger D, West D, Pitman T, *The Womanly Art of Breastfeeding.* 8th ed. London: Pinter and Martin; 2010. p152-153.

Chapter 17: Babies and Beds

1. Knowles R. *Why Babywearing Matters.* London: Pinter and Martin; 2016. p35.

2. Jackson D. *Three in a Bed.* London: Bloomsbury Publishing; 2003.

3. Brown A. *Breastfeeding Uncovered: Who Really Decides How We Feed Our Babies.* London: Pinter and Martin; 2016. p91&99-101.

4. Infant Sleep Information Source. Sleep Training. Durham: Durham University Parent-Infant Sleep Lab; 2015. Available from: https://www.dur.ac.uk/resources/isis.online/pdfs/ISIS_sleep training_2015.pdf [cited April 2017].

5. Pantley E. *The No-Cry Sleep Solution: Gentle Ways to Help Your Baby Sleep Through the Night.* New York: McGraw Hill; 2002.

6. Bolling K, Grant C, Hamlyn B, Thornton, A. Infant Feeding Survey 2005. London: The Information Centre for Health and Social Care; 2007.

7. Unicef, Co-sleeping and SIDS: A guide for health professionals. [Internet]. Unicef, 2017 Available from: https://www.unicef.org.uk/babyfriendly/wp-content/uploads/sites/2/2016/07/Co-sleeping-and-SIDS-A-Guide-for-Health-Professionals.pdf [cited June 19 2018].

8. NHS. Reducing the risk of sudden infant death syndrome (SIDS). [Internet]. Available from: https://www.nhs.uk/conditions/pregnancy-and-baby/reducing-risk-cot-death/ [cited 4 June 2018].

9. Gay CL, Lee KA, Lee S. Sleep patterns and fatigue in new mothers and fathers. *Biol Res Nurs.* 2004, Apr;5(4):311-318.

10. Unicef, Baby Friendly Initiative. Caring for your baby at night: A guide for Parents. London: Unicef UK Baby Friendly Initiative; 2017.

11. Ball H. Parent-infant bed-sharing behaviour : Effects of feeding type and presence of father. *Hum Nat.* 2006, Sep;17(3):301-318.

12. Wiessinger D, West D, Pitman T, *The Womanly Art of Breastfeeding.* 8th ed. London: Pinter and Martin; 2010. p227.

13. Henderson JMT, France KG, Owens JL, Blampied NM. Sleeping Through the Night: The Consolidation of Self-regulated Sleep Across the First Year of Life. *Pediatrics.* 2010, Nov;126(5):e1081-7.

Chapter 18: Sleep, or Lack Thereof

1. Jackson D. *Three in a Bed.* London: Bloomsbury Publishing;

2003.
2. Lee D, Willinger M, Petitti DB, Odouli R, Liu L, Hoffman HJ. Use of a dummy (pacifier) during sleep and risk of sudden infant death syndrome (SIDS): population based case-control study. *BMJ.* 2006, Jan;332(7532):18-22.
3. Rapley G, Murkett T. *Baby-led Breastfeeding.* London: Vermilion; 2012.
4. Pantley E. *The No-Cry Sleep Solution: Gentle Ways to Help Your Baby Sleep Through the Night.* New York: McGraw Hill; 2002.

Chapter 19: Why Bother Breastfeeding?

1. Palmer G. *The Politics of Breastfeeding.* London: Pinter and Martin; 2009. p37 & p91-97.
2. Duijts L, Jaddoe VWV, Hofman A, Moll HA. Prolonged and Exclusive Breastfeeding Reduces the Risk of Infectious Diseases in Infancy. 2010. *Pediatrics.* 2010, Jul;126(1):e18-25.
3. Monasta L, Batty GD, Cattaneo A, Lutje V, Ronfani L, Van Lenthe FJ, Brug J. Early-life determinants of overweight and obesity: a review of systematic reviews. *Obes Rev.* 2010, Oct;11 (10):695-708.
4. Pettit DJ. Forman MR, Hanson RL, Knowler WC, Bennett BH. Breastfeeding and the incidence of non insulin dependent diabetes mellitus in Pima Indians. *Lancet.* 1997, Jul;350(9072):166-168.
5. Kwan ML, Buffler PA, Abrams B, Kiley VA. Breastfeeding and the risk of childhood leukaemia: a meta-analysis. *Public Health Rep.* 2004, Nov-Dec;119(6):521-535.
6. Harman T, Wakeford A. *The Microbiome Effect.* London: Pinter and Martin; 2016. p56 & 94.
7. Chowdhury R, Sinha B, Saknar M, Teneja S, Bhandari N, Rollins N, Bahl R, Martines J. Breastfeeding and maternal health outcomes: a systematic review and meta-analysis. *Acta Paediatr.* 2015, Dec;104(467):96-113.
8. Schwarz EB, Ray, RM, Stuebe AM, Allison MA, Ness RB, Freiberg MS, Cauley JA. Duration of Lactation and Risk Factors

for Maternal Cardiovascular Disease. *Obstet Gynecol.* 2009, May;113(3):974-982.

9. Rapley G, Murkett T. *Baby-led Breastfeeding.* London: Vermilion; 2012. p136 138.

10. Uvnas Moberg, K. *The Oxytocin Factor.* London: Pinter and Martin; 2011. p126-127.

11. First Steps Nutrition Trust. Costs of Infant Milks. London: First Steps Nutrition Trust; 2018.

12. Kavanagh KF, Lou Z, Nicklas JC, Habibi MF, Murphy LT. Breastfeeding Knowledge, Attitudes, Prior Exposure, and Intent among Undergraduate Students. *J Hum Lact.* 2012, Nov;28(4):556-64.

13. Scott JA, Mostyn T. Women's experiences of breastfeeding in a bottlefeeding culture. *J Hum Lact.* 2003 Aug;19(3):270-7.

Chapter 20: Learning to Love Breastfeeding

1. Palmer G. *The Politics of Breastfeeding.* London: Pinter and Martin; 2009.

Chapter 21: Weaning

1. Grueger B, Canadian Paediatric Society. Weaning from the breast. *Paediatr Child Health.* 2013, Apr; 18(4):210-1.

2. Rapley G, Murkett T. *Baby-led Weaning.* London: Vermillion; 2008.

3. Renfrew MJ, Wallace LM, D'Souza L, McCormick F, Spiby H, Dyson L. The effectiveness of public health interventions to promote the duration of breastfeeding: systematic reviews of the evidence. London: National Institute for Health and Clinical Excellence; 2005. p5.

4. Wiessinger D, West D, Pitman T, *The Womanly Art of Breastfeeding.* 8th ed. London: Pinter and Martin; 2010. p93.

5. Evans, K. *The Food of Love.* Brighton: Myriad Editions; 2009.

p25.

6. Palmer G. *Complementary Feeding: Nutrition, Culture and Politics.* London: Pinter and Martin; 2011. p56.

7. Brown A. *Why Starting Solids Matters.* London: Pinter and Martin; 2017.

8. Castilho SD, Barros Filho ADA. The history of infant nutrition. *J Pediatria (Rio J)* . 2010, May/Jun;86(3);179-188.

9. Wilkinson PW, Davies DP. When and why are babies weaned? *BMJ.* 1978, June, 24;1(6128):1682-1683.

10. World Health Organization (WHO). Global strategy for infant and young child feeding. Geneva, WHO; 2003.

11. Kramer MS, Kakuma R. Optimal duration of exclusive breastfeeding. Geneva, World Health Organization; 2002.

12. Michaelson KF, Weaver L, Branca F, Robertson A. Feeding and Nutrition of Infants and Young Children: Guidelines for the WHO European Region with Emphasis on the former soviet Countries. Copenhagen; WHO Regional Publications. European Series, No. 87; 2003. p50.

13. Saarinen UM, Siimes MA. Iron Absorption from Breast Milk, Cow's Milk and Iron-supplemented Formula: An Opportunistic Use of Changes in Total Body Iron Determined by Hemoglobin, Ferritin and Body Weight in 132 Infants. *Pediat. Res.* 1979, Mar;13(3):143-7.

14. First Steps Nutrition Trust. Infant milks: A simple guide to infant formula, follow-on formula and other infant milks. London: First Steps Nutrition Trust; 2018.

Chapter 22: Taking the Back Seat

1. Fredregill S, Fredregill R. *Everything You Need to Know About Breastfeeding.* Updated edition. Newton Abbott: David and Charles; 2004, p80.

2. Gupta A, Khanna K, Chattree S. Cup feeding:an alternative to bottle feeding in a neonatal intensive care unit. *J Trop Pediatr.* 1999, Apr;46(2):108-10.

Chapter 23: Real Food

1. Wiessinger D, West D, Pitman T, *The Womanly Art of Breastfeeding.* 8th ed. London: Pinter and Martin; 2010. p152-153.
2. Brown A. *Breastfeeding Uncovered: Who Really Decides How We Feed Our Babies.* London: Pinter and Martin; 2016. p82.

Chapter 24: How Long is too Long?

1. Dettwyler KA. When to Wean: Biological Versus Cultural Perspectives. *Clin Obstet Gynaecol.* 2004, Sep;47(3):712-723.
2. Konner M, Worthman C. Nursing Frequency, Gonadal Function and Birth Spacing among !Kung Hinter Gatherers. *Science.* 1980, Feb;207(4432):788-91.
3. Grueger B, Canadian Paediatric Society. Weaning from the breast. *Paediatr Child Health.* 2013, Apr; 18(4):210-1.
4. Rapley G, Murkett T. *Baby-led Breastfeeding.* London: Vermilion; 2012. p169-170.
5. Chang-Claude J, Eby N, Kiechle M, Becher H. Breastfeeding and breast cancer risk by age 50 among women in Germany. *Cancer Causes Control.* 2000, Sep;11(8) 687-95.
6. Wiklund PK, Xu L, Wang Q, Mikkola T, Lyytikäinen A, Völgyi E, Munukka E, Cheng SM, Alen M, Keinänen-Kiukaanniemi S, Cheng S. Lactation is associated with greater maternal bone size and bone strength later in life. *Osteoporos Int.* 2012, Jul;23(7):1939-45.
7. Collaborative Group on Hormonal Factors in Breast Cancer. Breast cancer and breastfeeding: collaborative reanalysis of individual data from 47 epidemiological studies in 30 countries, including 50302 women with breast cancer and 96973 women without the disease. *Lancet.* 2002, Jul 20;360:187-95.
8. Evans, K. *The Food of Love.* Brighton: Myriad Editions; 2009. p186-187.
9. Rees C. Thinking about children's attachments. *Arch Dis Child.*

2005, Oct;90(10):1058-1065.

10. Wiessinger D, West D, Pitman T, *The Womanly Art of Breastfeeding*. 8th ed. London: Pinter and Martin; 2010. p335.

11. Riordan J. *Breastfeeding and Human Lactation*. 3rd ed. Boston and London: Jones and Bartlett; 2004. p80.

12. Sharma V, Corpse CS. Case Study Revisiting the Association Between Breastfeeding and Postpartum Depression. *J Hum Lact.* 2008, Feb;24(1):77-9.

Chapter 25: The End of the Road

1. Flower, H. *Adventures in Tandem Nursing*. Schaumburg, IL: La Leche League International, Inc; 2003. p46-48.

Chapter 26: Contraception and Birth Spacing

1. McNeilly AS. Effects of lactation on fertility. *Br Med Bull.* 1979;35(2) 151-4.

2. Ramos R, Kennedy KI, Visness CM. Effectiveness of lactational amenorrhoea in prevention of pregnancy in Manila, the Philippines: non-comparative prospective trial. *BMJ.* 1996, Oct, 12;313(7062):909-12.

3. Flower, H. *Adventures in Tandem Nursing*. Schaumburg, IL: La Leche League International, Inc; 2003.

4. Wiessinger D, West D, Pitman T, *The Womanly Art of Breastfeeding*. 8th ed. London: Pinter and Martin; 2010.

5. Jones, W. Contraception and Breastfeeding. Paisley: The Breastfeeding Network; 2017. Available from: https://breastfeedingnetwork.org.uk/wp-content/dibm/contraception%20and%20breastfeeding.pdf [cited 17th January 2018].

6. Palmer G. *The Politics of Breastfeeding*. London: Pinter and Martin; 2009.

7. Moscone SR, Moore MJ. Breastfeeding during Pregnancy. *J*

Hum Lact. 1993, Jun;9(2):83-88.

Chapter 27: Take Two

1. Bronsteen R, Valice R, Lee W, Blackwell S, Balasubramaniam M, Comstock C. Effect of a low-lying placenta on delivery outcome. *Ultrasound Obstet Gynecol.* 2009, Feb;33(2):204-8.
2. Blott M, editor. *The Day-by-Day Pregnancy Book.* London: Dorling Kindersley; 2009. p470.

Chapter 28: The Christmas Baby

1. Downey CL, Bewley S. Historical perspectives on umbilical cord clamping and neonatal transition. *J R Soc Med.* 2012, Aug;105(8)325-329.

Chapter 29: Babywearing

1. Kirkilionis E. *A Baby Wants to be Carried: Everything You Need to Know About Baby Carriers and the Benefits of Babywearing* (O'Donoghue, K, Trans). Pinter and Martin 2014 (Original work published 1999).
2. Sears W, Sears M. *The Baby Book.* 2nd ed. London: Thorsons; 2005. p308-9.
3. Knowles R. *Why Babywearing Matters.* London: Pinter and Martin; 2016.
4. Davies M. The Baby Carrier: a Child's First Country. [internet] Wales: Lindsay Magazine; 7 May 2018. Available from www.lindsaymagazine.co/baby-carrier-childs-first-country/ [cited 4 Jun 2018].
5. Rabin DL, Barnett CR, Arnold WD, Freiberger RH, Brooks G. Untreated congenital hip disease: A study of the epidemiology,

natural history, and social aspects of the disease in a Navajo population. *Am J Public Health Nations Health.* 1965, Feb;55:SUPPL:1-44.

6. Price CT, Schwend RM. Improper swaddling a risk factor for developmental dysplasia. *AAP News.* 2011;32(9).

7. Sewell SJ. The history of children's and invalids' carriages. *J R Soc Arts.* 1923, Sep;71(3694) 716-728.

8. V&A. Baby's pram 1905. [Internet]. Available from: https://www.vam.ac.uk/moc/collections/babys-pram-1905/ [cited June 17 2018].

9. Palmer G. *The Politics of Breastfeeding.* London: Pinter and Martin; 2009. p59.

10. Conde-Aguledo A, Díaz-Rossello JL. Kangaroo mother care to reduce morbidity and mortality in low birth weight infants. *Cochrane Database Syst Rev.* 2016; (8):CD002771.

Chapter 30: Completion?

1. Flower, H. *Adventures in Tandem Nursing.* Schaumburg, IL: La Leche League International, Inc; 2003. p47.

Chapter 31: Third Time Lucky

1. NHS Choices. Signs that labour has begun. [Internet] Available from: https://www.nhs.uk/conditions/pregnancy-and-baby/labour-signs-what-happens/ [cited 19 June 2018].

2. Wiessinger D, West D, Pitman T, *The Womanly Art of Breastfeeding.* 8th ed. London: Pinter and Martin; 2010.

ABOUT THE AUTHOR

Emma Rosen and her husband have three adorable children and a mad dog.

Having graduated with a Bachelor's degree in marine biology, Emma embarked on a teaching career, whilst also studying a Master's degree in education.

Emma loves all things breastfeeding and volunteers as a peer supporter at a local breastfeeding support group. When she's not writing or chasing her children, Emma makes YouTube videos, stares at the sea and sings in a band.

Lightning Source UK Ltd.
Milton Keynes UK
UKHW04f1013120918
328728UK00002B/187/P